BRITISH MEDICAL BULLETIN

British Medical Bulletin is published four times each year, in January, April, July and October.

Subscriptions and single-copy orders should be sent to: Longman Group UK Ltd, PO Box 77, Harlow, Essex CM19 5BQ. Tel: 0279 623760

Subscription rates for 1991 are: £92 (UK) or £105.00/$168.00 (overseas)

Single copies will be available at £29.95 (UK) or £35.00/$56.00 (overseas)

NEXT ISSUE

Volume 47 No. 4   Postviral Fatigue Syndrome   *October 1991*

Scientific Editors: Peter Behan, David Goldberg, James Mowbray

GU00802488

BRITISH MEDICAL BULLETIN

VOLUME FORTY-SEVEN
1991

CHURCHILL LIVINGSTONE
EDINBURGH, LONDON, MELBOURNE,
NEW YORK AND TOKYO

CHURCHILL LIVINGSTONE
Medical Division of Longman Group UK Limited

Distributed in the United States of America by Churchill
Livingstone Inc., 1560 Broadway, New York, NY 10036, and
by associated companies, branches and representatives
throughout the world.

ISSN 0007-1420
ISBN 0-443-04491-0

CHURCHILL LIVINGSTONE, Medical Division of Longman Group U.K. Limited.
Typeset and printed by H Charlesworth & Co Ltd, Huddersfield

Distributed in the United States of America by Churchill Livingstone Inc., 1560 Broadway,
New York, NY 10036, and by associated companies, branches and representatives through-
out the world. This journal is indexed, abstracted and/or published online in the following
media: Current Contents, Scientific Serials Review, Excerpta Medica, USSR Academy of
Science, Biological Abstracts, UMI (Microform), BRS Colleague (full text), Index Medicus,
BIOSIS, NMLUIS, Adonis

© The British Council 1991

ISSN 0007-1420   ISBN 0-443-04491-0

British Medical Bulletin is published quarterly in January, April, July and October by
Churchill Livingstone c/o Mercury Airfreight International Ltd Inc, 2323 Randolph
Avenue, Avenel, New Jersey 07001. Subscription price is $168.00. Second Class Postage
paid at Rahway NJ Postmaster: Send address corrections to British Medical Bulletin
c/o Mercury Airfreight International Ltd Inc, 2323 Randolph Avenue, Avenel, New Jersey
07001.

PAIN
Mechanisms
and Management

Scientific Editors:
J C D Wells C J Woolf

1991 Vol. 47 No. 3

Dr J C D Wells chaired the committee which included Dr C J Woolf, Professor G W Hawkes and Dr C J Main that planned this number of the British Medical Bulletin. We are grateful for their help and particularly to Dr Wells and Dr Woolf who acted as Scientific Editors for the number.

British Medical Bulletin is published by Churchill Livingstone for The British Council, 10 Spring Gardens, London SW1A 2BN

British Medical Bulletin (1991) Vol. 47, No. 3, pp. i–iv
© The British Council 1991

Introduction

S Lipton
Pain Relief Research Foundation, Rice Lane, Liverpool

Pain is one of the most important human experiences, and also one of the most complex. The International Association for the Study of Pain has defined pain as:

'An unpleasant sensory and emotional experience associated with actual or potential tissue damage, or described in terms of such damage. Pain is always subjective. Each individual learns the application of the word through experiences related to injury in early life. It is unquestionably a sensation in a part of the body, but it is also unpleasant, and therefore also an emotional experience. Many people report pain in the absence of tissue damage or any likely patho-physiological cause; usually this happens for psychological reasons. There is no way to distinguish their experience from that due to tissue damage, if we take this subjective report.'

In spite of the importance of pain, and the fact that it is the presenting symptom in over 60% of patients' consultations with doctors, until recently the interest of doctors was confined to its value as an indication of physical disease, with little attention being paid to the complexities of cultural and psychological factors which influence its severity, and the way in which each individual copes with it. This issue goes a long way towards correlating the recent understanding of the basic science concepts of pain, and the way they tie up with pain syndromes observed clinically. The scientific editors have assembled a group of world-renowned experts from both the basic science and clinical aspects of the investigation and management of pain. This underlines the importance of meticulous research in the basic science fields being extrapolated into clinical observations with humans. This has certainly been the objective of the Pain Relief Research Foundation, the first national pain charity to be set up worldwide to look at the causes and treatment of pain in humans.[1] This institution, based in Liverpool but with donations coming in from far afield, has helped to promote the close liaison between basic scientists and clinicians.

Acute pain is of course often useful in notifying the presence of disease, but once cognisance has been taken of this by the doctor, then the pain needs to be relieved *per se*, whilst the underlying disease is treated. This is sometimes something which is not well taught at medical school, and something which junior doctors tend to forget in the urgency of their work and the knowledge that the pain may be self-limiting (e.g. patients waiting for appendicectomy, or post-operative pain).

Chronic pain rarely serves any biological function, and in general terms causes a great deal of human suffering and a very high cost to both the individual and the state. Many doctors find chronic pain sufferers difficult to treat, because of their tendency not to improve over long periods of time, and to resist all treatments offered. There is often a conflict when the doctor tells the patient that he is imagining his pain, which of course is not an appropriate statement for an experience which can be emotional.

The existence of chronic pain is constantly underestimated. In the United States, it is estimated that 3.3% of the population are permanently disabled due to pain. Data from the United Kingdom shows that 21% of normal people complain of backache over a one month period. In 1985 in the United Kingdom there were 330 000 hospital referrals a year for back pain, and 63 000 hospital in-patient treatments averaging 2 weeks. Of these patients, 60% had unspecified backache, which was still not diagnosed at the time of discharge. The cost in 1982 of back pain was £156 million to the British National Health Service. The loss of working days caused by back pain was 33.3 million.

A recent study of nearly 1000 patients attending a diabetic clinic showed that 25% had chronic pain.[2] Given that there are some 1 million diabetics throughout the United Kingdom, this suggests that 250 000 diabetics have pain, and certainly 26% of this number have never had any treatment for this pain. The mean duration of pain in this group was 5 years. *Herpes zoster* occurs in 4 out of every 1000 of the population per year. Of these, 75% are over 60, and at least half go on to develop post-herpetic neuralgia. This gives an estimate of 1.5 people per 1000 per year developing post-herpetic neuralgia. As on average these sufferers have pain for approximately 3 years, this gives a figure of 225 000 people suffering from post-herpetic neuralgia at any one time.[3]

Scarce wonder then that a recent survey identified over 11% of the population in the United Kingdom as suffering from chronic pain. Many of these patients were disabled by their pain, most had been given up by the medical profession, and some had had no treatment whatsoever for their pain. This does not mean that such treatments do not exist. Perusal of this issue will indicate the excellent and ongoing work involved in classifying and measuring pain, in understanding the underlying mechanisms and in the treatment of these mechanisms and the symptomatic management of the various different pain states. Unfortunately this treatment is only available to a minority of patients, because of the lack of resources available. Even though there are over 200 Pain Clinics in the United Kingdom, many of these have a very long waiting list, of up to 2 years, before the patient can be seen. Even when seen, many do not have an adequate number of in-patient beds and resources in order to further investigate and better treat these chronic pain sufferers.

The relief of cancer pain has come a long way along the road to improvement. Some 20 years ago, although the medical and surgical techniques were available to treat these patients, lack of informed knowledge amongst doctors prevented their appropriate referral and consequent successful treatment. This has now been largely remedied, not least by the efforts worldwide of the World Health Organisation, who have taken the relief of cancer pain as one of their priorities. However, much work still needs to be done, as although doctors in some countries are aware of what treatments are available and are successful, those treatments are just not accessible. In Turkey and the Far East, it has proved very difficult to obtain morphine as an oral medication, also in South America, all of this because of fears of dependency. In India, where the drug is theoretically available, in practice it is expensive and not obtainable for the vast majority of the population in rural communities. Whilst work continues to be carried out in the Western world in the way of refining treatments and reducing side-effects, the priority in much of the third world is to make sure that facilities for such treatment exist.

A recent paper by the Royal College of Surgeons indicated the unsatisfactory state of affairs with regard to management of acute pain, particularly post-operative. The chapter by Justins & Richardson indicates how much can be done to alleviate acute pain, but even in the United Kingdom this is not always done at a satisfactory level. Hopefully this knowledge of the current state of affairs will stimulate the setting-up of acute pain services, which are probably best linked through existing pain relief teams and Pain Relief Clinics.

Thus it will be seen that, despite the knowledge obtained from this book, further progress will require increased health education amongst pain sufferers, and also education of those key personnel who hold the purse strings which will enable a sufficient amount of money to be used in an appropriate fashion. There is still an urgent need for increased resources to allow research into all aspects of pain, and there needs to be a great increase in resources to apply the currently known methods of treatment. In the meantime, this book gives an update of the state-of-the-art understanding of various important pain mechanisms, and in the most appropriate current management of many important forms of pain.

REFERENCES

1 Lipton S, Jones ARJ. The Pain Relief Foundation (PRF) researches human intractable Pain — Assessment, biochemistry, physiological pathways and treatment. Pain 1987; (Supp 4): S372
2 Chan AW, MacFarlane IA, Bowsher D, Wells JCD, Griffiths K, Bessex C. Chronic pain in patients with diabetes mellitus. Comparison with a non-diabetic population. The Pain Clinic 1990; 3: 147–159
3 Harding SP, Lipton JR, Wells JCD. Natural history of *Herpes Zoster* opthalmicus: predictors of post-herpetic neuralgia and ocular involvement. Br J Ophthalmol 1987; 71(5): 353–8

British Medical Bulletin (1991) Vol. 47, No. 3, pp. 523–533
© The British Council 1991

Generation of acute pain: Central mechanisms

C J Woolf
Department of Anatomy and Developmental Biology, University College London, London, UK

Pain can either be 'nociceptor-mediated', produced as a consequence of the activation of high threshold nociceptors, or 'A-fibre mediated', resulting from the activation of low threshold $A\beta$ afferent fibres. Under normal circumstances nociceptor mediated pain only occurs in response to high intensity noxious stimuli. Following peripheral tissue injury the inflammatory reaction generates a complex set of chemical signals that alter the transduction properties of nociceptors such that they can be activated by low intensity stimuli, the phenomenon of peripheral sensitization. Pain in this circumstance is still nociceptor mediated but can be generated by low intensity or innocuous stimuli. The nociceptive input to the spinal cord in these circumstances however produces activity-dependent alterations in the response properties of neurones in the dorsal horn. This means that they begin to repond to normal inputs, including that generated by $A\beta$ low threshold afferents, in an abnormal and exaggerated way. This is the phenomenon of central sensitization. Because afferent inputs can provoke prolonged alterations within the central nervous system, optimal treatment of acute pain states should be directed both at abolishing peripheral sensitization and to preventing the establishment of central sensitization. The latter involves the strategy of pre-emptive analgesia.

Pain, like all conscious sensations, is the culmination of complex sensory processing within the highest levels of the nervous system.

The key to understanding the pathogenesis of pain lies not in establishing the operation of these high order centres but in identifying the precise nature of the input signals that trigger the perception of this and not other sensory experiences. In order to begin to do this it is useful to consider some general aspects of painful sensations. In many respects pain at first may seem to resemble other somatosensations in having qualities or attributes that can be referred directly to an initiating stimulus in the periphery. An example of this is the common use of the term a 'painful stimulus', which is essentially a prediction that a certain type of input will elicit pain. The expectation of pain in this case is a recognition that similar stimuli in the past have invariably produced pain. Because this experience is shared by most people we tend to use a mental 'shorthand' that equates a particular class of stimuli with the sensation of pain. Intuitively this analysis would seem to imply that the production of pain is simply the process whereby certain stimuli, 'painful stimuli', are converted to signals, 'pain signals', in specific sensory nerve fibres, 'pain fibres', and that this specific 'pain' information is conserved within the central nervous system. The only encoding that such a 'pain' pathway need perform would be that related to intensity, duration and location of the 'painful' stimulus.

The treatment of pain, if this model were correct would simply be a matter of finding the most effective way of interrupting the 'pain system' at some point, either in the periphery or within the central nervous system. The view that pain is a specific sensation generated by specific inputs has dominated contemporary neurophysiology and clinical practice until very recently because it is simple and because it is in keeping with our own acute pain experiences. That such an analysis is inadequate can readily be appreciated however, if we look at the relationship between stimulus and response that occurs in clinical pain. Here a direct connection between the sensory experience of pain and a unique class of stimuli is lost. Instead we have a characteristic pattern of unpleasant sensations, ranging from discomfort to agony, that are typically generated by everyday manoeuvres such as walking, moving, coughing and touching. There are no longer distinct 'painful' stimuli instead patients often find that their pain is spontaneous or elicited by what normally would be regarded as totally innocuous or 'non-painful' stimuli. Whether we consider the pain associated with acute inflammation or that resulting from nerve injury we are clearly dealing with something qualitatively quite different from the acute pain that results from a transient high intensity or noxious stimulus.

Essentially we need to recognize that there are two separate pain phenomena. The first is the pain that results under normal circumstances only from intense or potentially damaging noxious stimuli activating nociceptors (high threshold sensory receptors), which can be termed physiological pain, and the second is the pain that results from low intensity or innocuous stimuli in clinical situations and which has been called pathological pain.[1,2] Physiological pain is highly localized and if no tissue damage is produced, transient. This is the pain we perceive in response to firm pressure or pinch, excessive heat or cold, chemical irritants, and mild abrasions to the skin. Its role is simple but important, to inform the body of potential danger, which is why it is so highly correlated with the initiation of the flexion withdrawal response.[3] This pain has distinct mechanical, thermal and chemical thresholds and its amplitude is related to the intensity of the stimulus in a measurable way. The reason for this is that it is a pain that is driven by functionally specialized nociceptor afferent fibres which encode aspects of noxious stimuli related to their modality, intensity, duration and location.[4] Physiological pain can therefore be considered to constitute a 'nociceptor-mediated' pain (Fig. 1).

Pathological pain in contrast is that pain that arises following tissue or nerve damage. It is characterized by a disruption of normal sensory mechanisms so that the pain can occur in the absence

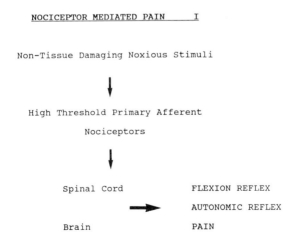

Fig. 1 A model of the neural mechanisms that operate to produce 'physiological' pain by the activation of nociceptors by high intensity peripheral stimuli.

of a clear stimulus, in response to innocuous stimuli, and in an exaggerated and prolonged fashion to noxious stimuli. All three examples represent an increase in the sensitivity of the sensory system, the phenomenon of nociceptive sensitization, with a reduction in pain thresholds (allodynia) an amplification of responsiveness (hyperalgesia) and prolonged post-stimulus sensations (hyperpathia). This pain in its acute form, usually associated with tissue damage and inflammation—inflammatory pain, has a protective function. The increased sensitivity of the system promotes recuperation and repair by minimizing further injury by avoiding **all** contact rather than just preventing contact with noxious stimuli. In its chronic form, usually associated with nerve damage-neuropathic pain, the pain seems to have lost any adaptive function and is truly pathological.

Nociceptive sensitization results from changes in the peripheral terminals of primary afferent nociceptors (peripheral sensitization) and from changes in the response properties of neurones in the spinal cord (central sensitization). The aim of this chapter is to demonstrate that the recognition that alterations in the central nervous system have a major role in the production of pathological pain states has led to a new approach or strategy for the treatment of pain; pre-emptive analgesia.

Nociceptor-mediated pain

Physiological pain is the consequence of the activation of nociceptive afferents by high intensity noxious stimuli (Fig. 1). Once the threshold of these afferents is exceeded and an afferent barrage in Aδ and C afferents to the spinal cord is generated three different responses can occur. The first is the activation of flexor motor neurons producing the flexion withdrawal reflex. The second, acting at spinal and supraspinal levels, is the activation of sympathetic preganglionic neurones producing a general autonomic response (changes in heart rate and blood pressure) and a segmental response (changes in local blood flow, piloerection and sweating). The third response is the generation of the sensation of pain and of pain-like behaviour (coordinated escape responses, vocalization etc.).

Pathological pain can be produced by nociceptors and, unlike physiological pain, by large myelinated A fibres. The mechanisms and site of changes that operate to produce nociceptor and A-fibre mediated pathological pain are different. The nociceptor mediated pain in this situation is generated by nociceptors whose response properties and sensitivity are altered (Fig. 2). These changes, constituting **peripheral sensitization**, result from tissue damage and the consequent inflammatory response.[5,6] The elements contributing to the inflammation include a non-neurogenic component; directly damaged cells which release their intracellular contents, inflammatory cells including mast cells, macrophages, lymphocytes and polymorphonuclear cells releasing cytokines, and a neurogenic component comprising somatosensory afferent and postganglionic sympathetic efferent terminals.[7,8] The somatosensory afferents in addition to transferring electrical signals to the CNS also have a motor function, releasing transmitters such as substance P and CGRP (calcitonin gene related peptide) that act on inflammatory cells, smooth muscle cells and endothelial cells producing vasodilatation and the extravasation of plasma proteins as well as acting on inflammatory cells.[9,10] The sympathetic boutons appear to contribute to this both directly and indirectly by releasing chemicals that potentiate the actions of some of the inflammatory mediators on afferents and inflammatory cells and by changing the microcirculation.[11] One consequence of these complex cellular interactions is the release of a 'sensitizing soup' containing neuropeptides, histamine, 5-HT, potassium ions, bradykinin and arachidonic acid metabolites which alter the transduction properties of some high threshold nociceptors[12] (*see* Rang

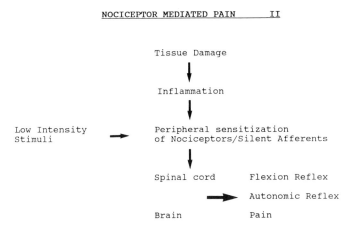

Fig. 2 A model illustrating how alterations in the sensitivity of the peripheral terminals of nociceptors produced by inflammatory mediators, peripheral sensitization, can result in pain that is nociceptor mediated but activated by low intensity or innocuous stimuli.

et al., this issue). This means that low intensity stimuli which would not normally activate nociceptors begin to do so and therefore a 'nociceptor-mediated pain' generated by low intensity stimuli results (Fig. 2).

A recent important finding is that under normal circumstances a substantial number of afferents (10–40%) are silent, failing to respons to stimuli directed to skin or deep tissues. Following inflammation, however, some of the chemicals released activate these afferent terminals so that they now begin to respond to mechanical or thermal stimuli. An example of this is that of a subpopulation of joint afferents which don't respond to the normal range of flexion and extension but begin to do so following an experimental arthritis.[13]

A-fibre mediated pain

The capacity of the peripheral terminals of primary afferent nociceptors to become sensitized is clearly of considerable importance in many acute pain states and indeed may be the exclusive cause of pathological pain in certain rare conditions.[14] However it is not the sole explanation for the generation of clinical pains. The reason for this can be illustrated by the following two experimental observations. The first is that although cutaneous injury produces a considerable degree of mechanical hypersensitivity at the site of the injury in man[15] and in animals,[16] there are few reports of sensitization of high threshold mechanoreceptor afferents.[5] Most examples of cutaneous peripheral sensitization are to thermal stimuli.[5,6] The second is that cutaneous injury produces two zones of hyperalgesia one at the site of injury, primary hyperalgesia, and one in the surrounding uninjured tissue, secondary hyperalgesia.[5] Although there is considerable mechanosensitivity in the zone of secondary hyperalgesia no studies have been able to demonstrate changes in nociceptors in this region.[15] This implies that some component of the altered sensitivity to stimuli that accompanies peripheral tissue injury must be the result of an abnormal central response to inputs that normally only produce innocuous sensations. In other words clinical pain involves a transformation from a situation where only nociceptors can drive the nervous system to produce pain to one where Aβ afferents can (Fig. 3).

Under normal circumstances the activation of low threshold Aβ afferents by tactile stimuli, pressure to deep tissue, movements of joints etc. does not produce pain. How can they begin to do so

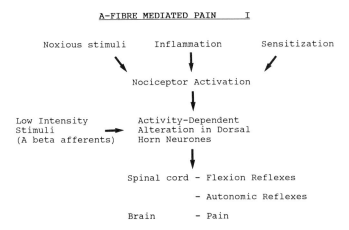

Fig. 3 A model demonstrating that nociceptor activation, by triggering alterations in the response properties of neurones in the spinal cord, the phenomenon of central sensitization, enable A-fibre inputs to begin to produce pain, something they never normally do.

under pathological circumstances. The answer lies in the capacity of neurones in the dorsal horn of the spiral cord to undergo prolonged alterations in their response properties, the phenomenon of **central sensitization**.[2] Figure 3 illustrates how the activation of nociceptors directly by noxious stimuli or following their sensitization, by low intensity stimuli, produce activity-dependent alterations in dorsal horn neurones such that they begin to respond in an abnormal or exaggerated way to Aβ afferent inputs. Essentially what happens is that cells whose predominant drive under normal circumstances is from nociceptors begin to be activated by Aβ afferents, and multiconvergent cells get an even larger A-fibre input.[17] These afferents can now evoke flexion withdrawal reflexes, autonomic responses and pain sensations.

What are the nature of the changes produced by nociceptor afferents in dorsal horn neurones and how do these changes enable an aberrant convergence of inputs to occur? The answer to the first question appears to be related to the capacity of small diameter afferents (Aδ and C) and not the large Aβ afferents to produce slow synaptic potentials in spinal neurones.[18] The duration of classical fast excitatory postsynaptic potentials is 10–20 ms. Small diameter afferents produce slow potentials that last for up to 20 s. Two mechanisms operate to produce these long lasting depolarizations. The first is the release by nociceptor afferents of neuropeptides (such as substance P, neurokinin A, CGRP etc.) which have long lasting effects. The second is that dorsal horn neurones possess a form of excitatory amino acid receptor, the N-methyl-D-aspartate acid (NMDA) receptor that acts to prolong the duration of synaptic potentials.[18] This receptor-ion channel complex has an important property. At normal resting membrane potentials the ion channel is blocked by magnesium ions and therefore the excitatory amino acid glutamate or a similar compound binding to the NMDA receptor will produce no effect. However, if the membrane is depolarized either by one of the other excitatory amino acid receptors or by a neuropeptide, the magnesium block is removed from the ion channel and sodium and calcium ions enter the cell producing a further depolarization.[19] The long duration of the slow potentials enables a remarkable degree of temporal summation. Provided the slow potential has not returned to baseline levels, a second input will summate with the first and produce an incrementing response. The frequency of stimuli required to produce such a cumulatively increasing depolarization is low, only between 0.5 and 2.0 Hz.[18] Once the depolarization is established by a brief train of Aβ or C fibre inputs it persists for several minutes and during this period the response of the cell to all inputs including Aβ afferents is augmented. These changes are not sufficient to account for the prolonged central facilitation that have been shown experimentally to occur following brief noxious stimuli or the electrical stimulation of C-afferents.[20,21] Here we need to invoke metabolic changes induced by the afferent inputs in the dorsal horn neurones. The NMDA receptor-ion channel as already mentioned can allow calcium ions to enter the cells. In this direct way second messenger—protein kinase systems can be activated. Alternatively protein kinases could be activated by afferent transmitters binding to G-protein linked receptors. Histochemical studies have provided evidence for an NMDA mediated activation of protein kinase activity in the dorsal horn.[22] Protein kinases by phosphorylating a variety of target proteins, ion channels, receptors, enzymes etc. could produce changes in the properties of the cells that long outlast the initiating stimulus. Even longer lasting changes have the potential to be produced by brief afferent inputs because such inputs can alter gene-expression. This has most dramatically been demonstrated for the immediate-early genes[23] but also for the endogenous kappa agonist dynorphin.[24] Therefore the machinery is in place to enable the transformation of brief inputs of electrical activity in certain sensory input pathways into long lasting changes in neurones in the CNS.

The reason why an increase in the excitability of dorsal horn neurones changes sensory processing, such that Aβ afferents begin to produce pain, is because the receptive field properties of dorsal horn neurones contain both suprathreshold and subliminal components.[25] The suprathreshold component manifests as action potential discharge while the subliminal component comprises the generation of subthreshold synaptic potentials. These subthreshold inputs are found in the majority of dorsal horn neurons.[25] An increase in synaptic efficacy or membrane excitability resulting from a brief nociceptive afferent input, by converting the subthreshold input to suprathreshold responses will produce an increase in response to standard stimuli, an expansion of the size of receptive fields and a reduction in threshold. This has been demonstrated directly, including the conversion of 'nociceptive specific' cells into multireceptive cells which respond to innocuous as well as noxious inputs.[17]

The changes in the peripheral and central nervous system that have been described in this Chapter relate specifically to acute pain mechanisms. However the same sort of general category of changes occur following peripheral nerve injury with the generation of an A-fibre mediated pain, which in this case may be due both to an altered responsiveness of central neurones and changes in synaptic circuitry (Fig. 4; *see* Devon & Wall, this issue.)

Clinical implications of central sensitization

The capacity of nociceptive afferents to induce a state of central sensitization has important consequences for pain management. Effectively it means that attempts should be made to prevent the initiation of central sensitization if possible, and once it has been produced, to recognize that a treatment directed purely at preventing nociceptor activation in the periphery is likely to be inadequate on its own if the nervous system remains in an abnormal state, because it can be driven by low threshold afferents. This can be translated in clinical practice to strategies aimed at preventing the afferent barrage generated by tissue injury from reaching the central nervous system. Obviously this can best be realized for elective surgical procedures with a regional local anaesthetic block before the surgeon touches the patient with a scalpel blade. In a recent trial comparing such treatment with conventional general anaesthetic, the postoperative demand for analgesics and pain were significantly reduced.[26] A similar reduction in postoperative pain

A-FIBRE MEDIATED PAIN   II

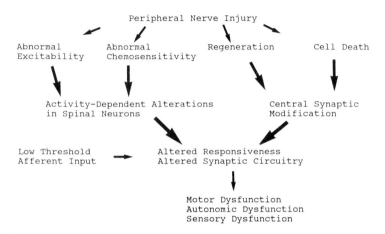

Fig. 4 The pain associated with peripheral nerve injury may have an A-fibre mediated component that is the result both of activity dependent changes in spinal neurones and of an altered synaptic circuitry consequent on degenerative and regenerative changes produced by the nerve injury.

has also been observed in patients given opiate premedication.[27] The best treatment for pain appears to be therefore that treatment is initiated before the pain is experienced.

REFERENCES

1 Woolf CJ. Physiological, inflammatory and neuropathic pain. Adv Tech Stand Neurosurg 1987; 15: 39–62
2 Woolf CJ. Recent advances in the pathophysiology of acute pain. Br J Anaesth 1989; 63: 139–146
3 Willer JC. Comparative study of perceived pain and nociceptive flexion reflex in man. Pain 1979; 3: 69–80
4 Burgess PR, Perl ER. Cutaneous mechanoreceptors and nociceptors. In: Iggo A, ed. Handbook of sensory physiology, somatosensory system, Vol. 2. Heidelberg; Springer, 1973
5 Bessou P, Perl ER. Response of cutaneous sensory units with unmyelinated fibres to noxious stimuli. J Neurophysiol 1969; 32: 1025–1043
6 Campbell JN, Meyer RA, LaMotte RH. Sensitization of myelinated nociceptive afferents that innervate monkey hand. J Neurophysiol 1979; 42: 1669–1679
7 LaMotte RH, Thalhammer JG, Robinson CJ. Peripheral neural correlates of magnitude of cutaneous pain and hyperalgesia: A comparison of neural events in monkey with sensory judgements in human. J Neurophysiol 1983; 50: 1–26
8 Raja S, Meyer JN, Meyer RA. Peripheral mechanisms of somatic pain. Anesthesiology 1988; 68: 571–590
9 Brain SD, Williams TJ. Inflammatory oedema induced by synergism between

calcitonin gene-related peptide and mediators of increased vascular permeability. Br J Pharmacol 1985; 86: 855–860

10 Otten U, Erhard P, Peck R. Nerve growth factor induces growth and differentiation of human B lymphocytes. Proc Natl Acad Sci USA 1989; 86: 10059–10063

11 Levine JD, Taiwo YO, Collins SD, Tam JK. Noradrenaline hyperalgesia is mediated through interaction with sympathetic postganglionic neurone terminals rather than activation of primary afferent nociceptors. Nature 1986; 323: 158–160

12 Lang E, Novak A, Reeh PW, Handwerker HO. Chemosensitivity of fine afferents from rat skin in vitro. J Neurophysiol 1990; 63: 887–901

13 Grigg P, Schiable HG, Schmidt RF. Mechanical sensitivity of group III and IV from the posterior articular nerve in normal and inflamed knee. J Neurophysiol 1986; 55: 635–643

14 Ochoa J. The newly recognized painful ABC syndrome: thermographic aspects. Thermology 1986; 2: 65–107

15 Raja S, Campbell JN, Meyer RA. Evidence for different mechanisms of primary and secondary hyperalgesia following heat injury to the glabrous skin. Brain 1984; 107: 1179–1188

16 Woolf CJ. Long term alterations in the excitability of the flexion reflex produced by peripheral tissue injury in the chronic decerebrate rat. Pain 1984; 18: 325–343

17 Woolf CJ, King AE. Dynamic alterations in the cutaneous mechanosensitive receptive fields of dorsal horn neurons in the rat spinal cord. J Neurosci 1990, (In press)

18 Thompson SWN, King AE, Woolf CJ. Activity-dependent changes in rat ventral horn neurones in vitro; summation of prolonged afferent evoked postsynaptic depolarizations produce a d-APV sensitive windup. Eur J Neurosci 1990; 2: 638–649

19 Mayer ML, Westbrook G, Guthrie PB. Voltage-dependent block by Mg^{2+} of NMDA responses in spinal cord neurones. Nature 1984; 309: 261–263

20 Woolf CJ. Evidence for a central component of postinjury pain hypersensitivity. Nature 1983; 308: 686–688

21 Woolf CJ, Wall PD. The relative effectiveness of C primary afferent fibres of different origins in evoking a prolonged facilitation of the flexor reflex in the rat. J Neurosci 1986; 6: 1433–1443

22 Woolf CJ. Excitatory amino acids increase glycogen phosphorylase activity in the rat spinal cord. Neurosci Lett 1987; 73: 209–214

23 Hunt SP, Pini A, Evan G. Induction of C-fos-like protein in spinal cord neurones following sensory stimulation. Nature 1987; 328: 632–634

24 Iadarola MJ, Brady LS, Draisci G, Dubner R. Enhancement of dynorphin gene expression in spinal cord following experimental inflammation: stimulus specificity, behavioural parameters and opioid receptor binding. Pain 1988; 35: 313–326

25 Woolf CJ, King AE. Subthreshold components of the receptive fields of dorsal horn neurones in the rat. J Neurophysiol 1989; 62: 907–916

26 Tverskoy M, Cozacov C, Ayache M, Bradley EL, Kissin I. Postoperative pain after inguinal herniorrhaphy with different types of anesthesia. Anesth Analg 1990; 70: 29–35

27 McQuay HJ, Carroll D, Moore RA. Postoperative orthopaedic pain—the effect of opiate premedication and local anaesthetic blocks. Pain 1988; 33: 291–295

British Medical Bulletin (1991) Vol. 47, No. 3, pp. 534–548
© The British Council 1991

Chemical activation of nociceptive peripheral neurones

H P Rang
S Bevan
A Dray
Sandoz Institute for Medical Research, London, UK

In inflammation, non-neuronal cells produce a variety of chemical mediators that act on nociceptive neurones. Ultimately, the discharge of these neurones is controlled by the activity of membrane ion channels. Some chemical mediators (e.g. ATP, protons, 5-hydroxytryptamine) act on receptors that are linked directly to ion channels. Other mediators (e.g. bradykinin) act indirectly through receptors linked to second messenger systems and in this way modulate the activity of ion channels and either activate or sensitize the neurones. The eicosanoids, which are produced by a variety of cell types, have important intra- and inter-cellular roles in nociception. The interactions between neurones and non-neuronal cells are likely to be complex as some types of non-neuronal cells express receptors for sensory neuropeptides (substance P). Recent studies also suggest that cytokines and growth factors can have long term effects on nociceptive neurone function.

Excitation of small-diameter sensory nerve fibres in the periphery by adequate stimuli is well-known to elicit pain. The physiological characteristics of these nociceptive fibres have been extensively studied.[1-3] The nociceptive fibres can be divided into two main groups, of which the largest is the C-polymodal nociceptors (C-PMNs). These are abundant, non-myelinated sensory fibres, which constitute the majority of the fibres in many sensory nerves. Polymodal nociceptors respond to all three types of noxious stimulus—namely thermal, mechanical and chemical. This class of sensory neurones is exceptional also in the abundance of neuropeptides that they contain and release during activity. They also show the property of sensitization following repeated heat stimulation, a property which may be important in relation to the state of hyperalgesia that follows tissue injury. The second main group of nociceptive neurones comprises fine myelinated (Aδ) fibres known as A-mechano-heat (AMH) fibres. As their name implies, these respond mainly to mechanical and thermal stimulation in the noxious range; they also respond, though less strongly than the C-PMNs, to chemical stimuli such as bradykinin and capsaicin. A proportion of these neurones also express neuropeptides. Many studies have provided evidence for subdivisions of these two main categories of nociceptors, but the details evidently vary according to tissue and species.

Nociceptive neurones show a further important characteristic, namely plasticity, whereby their responsiveness to stimuli can vary, particularly in the presence of chemical mediators of inflammation. One aspect of this phenomenon is that of sensitization, which is a factor in the mechanism of primary hyperalgesia, a lowering of the threshold to pain localized to an area of tissue damage. This is distinct from secondary hyperalgesia which involves a lowered pain threshold in areas beyond the site of injury, and may be of greater functional importance. Secondary hyperalgesia is known to occur primarily through adaptive changes in central synaptic transmission, rather than in peripheral sensory nerve terminals (*see* Woolf, this issue).

In this article, we concentrate on the various types of chemical sensitivity that characterize nociceptive neurones. There seems little doubt that such chemosensitivity is an important factor in many forms of inflammatory pain, and it may also provide a rational basis for the development of new kinds of analgesic drugs.

ACTIONS OF CHEMICAL MEDIATORS

The control of the discharge of nociceptive neurones by chemical mediators depends ultimately on the effects of these mediators on membrane ion channels (Fig. 1). These may be **directly** coupled to membrane receptors for specific substances (receptor-gated ion channels), or may be controlled **indirectly** through intracellular second messengers. The effects of chemical mediators acting in either of these ways may be to elicit discharges directly, or to enhance the excitatory effects of other stimuli. At higher levels of organization, some mediators may act at other parts of the neurone, for example to control, at the gene-transcription level, the expression of receptor proteins or ion channels, or their transport to nerve terminals; they may also act to control the release of mediators by other cells. Examples of agents that affect nociceptor function at these different levels are shown in Table 1 and the main mechanisms are summarized in Figures 1 and 2. In some cases (e.g. kainate, $GABA_A$, $GABA_B$), these receptors do not appear to play a role in peripheral nociception and are probably important for mechanisms operating at the presynaptic afferent terminals. A brief overview of some of the principal mediators and mechanisms based on current but incomplete knowledge will now be presented.

PATHOPHYSIOLOGICAL ACTIVATORS AND SENSITIZERS

Protons

Inflammatory exudates are usually acidic, and anecdotal observations confirm the painfulness of acidic solutions applied to exposed tissues. Protons have an excitatory effect on many neurones, producing a brief depolarization that inactivates within a few seconds.[4] In some sensory neurones, however, this response is followed by a maintained depolarization, associated with an increased ionic conductance and an inward current.[5] These neurones are also sensitive to capsaicin, which indicates that they are likely to be nociceptive. The responses to protons and capsaicin show many similarities which raises the possibility that H^+ is the endogenous activator of a membrane ion channel associated with a capsaicin receptor. However, the binding sites for protons and

Table 1 Molecular sites of action of mediators that affect nociceptive neurones. Some agents have no obvious, physiologically relevant, peripheral actions and probably exert their effect at the central terminals of the afferent neurones; these are not discussed in the text

Site	↑ or ↓ in excitability	Examples (receptor type)
Ion channels	↑	Capsaicin, H^+, ATP (P2), 5-HT (3), kainate
	↓	Local anaesthetics, GABA (A)
Receptors linked to 2nd messengers	↑	Bradykinin (B2), Eicosanoids, 5HT (1), Histamine (1)
	↓	Opiates (??), somatostatin, adrenoceptor agonists, GABA (B)

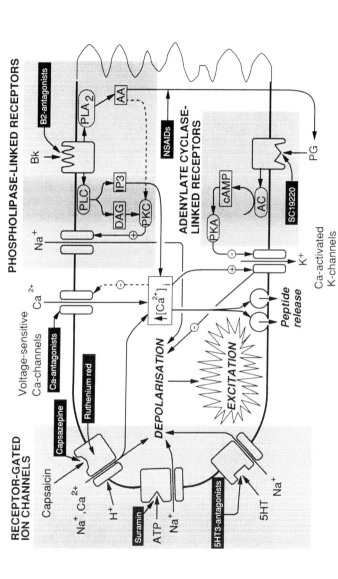

Fig. 1 Simplified scheme showing some of the intracellular processes involved in the control of the excitability of nociceptive nerve terminals. Several receptor-mediated processes have been omitted for clarity, such as the inhibitory effects of opioids (which act partly by opening K^+-channels and partly by inhibiting Ca^{2+}-channel opening, through inhibition of adenylate cyclase) and GABA (which acts partly by opening Cl^--channels and partly by inhibiting Ca^{2+}-channel opening)

Abbreviations: PLC, phospholipase C; PLA_2, phospholipase A_2; DAG, diacylglycerol; IP3, inositol-1,4,5-trisphosphate; PKC, protein kinase C; AA, arachidonic acid; cAMP, cyclic adenosine monophosphate; AC, adenylate cyclase; PKA, cAMP-dependent protein kinase; Bk, bradykinin; 5HT, 5-hydroxytryptamine; NSAIDs, non-steroidal anti-inflammatory drugs. SC19220 is a PG antagonist (see Ref 49).

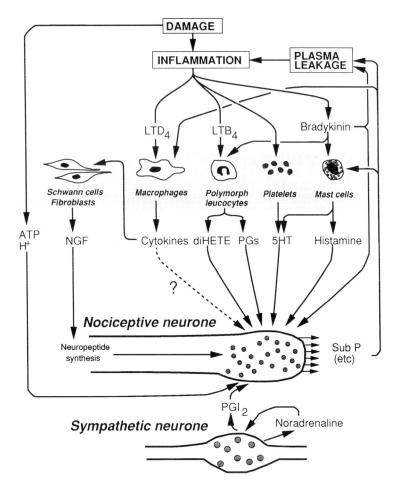

Fig. 2 Simplified scheme showing some of the local mediators that may act on nociceptive nerve terminals under conditions of tissue damage and inflammation, as discussed in text. The postulated interaction between sympathetic and nociceptive neurones is discussed in detail by MacMahon (this issue)

Abbreviations: LTD_4, leukotriene D_4; LTB_4, leukotriene B_4; NGF, nerve growth factor; diHETE, dihydroxy-eicosatetraenoic acid; PGs, prostaglandins E & $F_{2\alpha}$; 5HT, 5-hydroxytryptamine.

capsaicin may well be distinct since the effect of protons is resistant to the specific capsaicin antagonist capsazepine (see below).

Adenosine triphosphate

ATP is a ubiquitous component of cells, present at millimolar levels, so that tissue damage is likely to release large amounts in the vicinity of sensory nerve endings. Intradermal injection of ATP produces a sharp but transient pain. In rat sensory neurones ATP at micromolar concentrations excites a subpopulation of neurones and elicits an increase in cation permeability by direct activation of an ion channel.[6,7] This effect appears to be blocked by certain P_2-receptor antagonists such as suramin. The characteristics of the ATP-activated channel are unusual in that large organic cations such as tetraethylammonium are permeant, and the channel does not discriminate between monovalent cations such as Na^+, K^+, Cs^+. The channels are also permeant to divalent Ca^{2+} ions.

Interestingly, ATP receptors are also present on macrophages. Their activation may result in the release of various cytokines and prostanoids that are known to sensitize sensory neurones as discussed below.

5-Hydroxytryptamine

5HT can be released from blood platelets and mast-cells during tissue damage and can either sensitize or directly activate nociceptors. In studies on human blister base the pain evoked by 5HT, is mild and transient. However, application of 5HT to the blister base at a concentration insufficient to cause pain produces a marked sensitization to subsequent administration of bradykinin. Interestingly the sensitizing effect of 5-HT is inhibited by the $5HT_3$-receptor antagonist ICS 205.930.[8] This antagonist also reduced the hyperalgesia, but not the oedema, associated with carageenan-induced inflammation, suggesting that 5HT is a mediator of inflammatory hyperalgesia.[9] However, the possibility that other subtypes of 5HT receptors, such as the novel $5HT_4$ receptor, which is also blocked by ICS 205.930[10], are involved in hyperalgesia, cannot at present be excluded.

Some subtypes of 5HT receptors have been shown to couple with various second messenger systems. Thus $5HT_{1c}$ and $5HT_2$ receptors activate membrane phospholipase C, whereas other $5HT_1$ receptor subtypes and $5HT_4$ receptors are coupled to adenylate cyclase. $5HT_3$ receptors however appear to be directly linked to ion channels.[11] This receptor is present on capsaicin-sensitive sensory neurones where 5HT and the $5HT_3$ ligand, 2-methyl-5HT, activate an inward current. This effect of $5HT_3$-receptor activation is sensitive to ICS 205-930.[12] Thus 5-HT receptors on sensory neurones are coupled to ligand-gated sodium channels, and this mechanism may be responsible for the direct pain-producing effect of 5-HT. 5HT can have other effects on sensory neurones, such as modulation of voltage-gated Ca currents[13] and inhibition of a slow hyperpolarizing after-potential.[14] These effects, which are mediated by pathways involving second messengers, rather than by direct channel activation, may be involved in 5-HT-induced nociceptor sensitization.

Bradykinin

This nonapeptide, produced by cleavage of high molecular weight kininogens following protease activation at sites of tissue injury, is one of the most potent pain-producing substances present in inflammatory exudates and damaged tissue. Although bradykinin activates sensory neurones, it also exerts a variety of effects on many other cell types: it is mitogenic, it stimulates secretion, contracts smooth muscle, stimulates endothelial cell activity and frequently mobilizes cellular arachidonic acid, leading to prostanoid formation. It is difficult to identify the relative contributions of these various actions to the pain-producing and pro-inflammatory effects of bradykinin. The synthesis and release of eicosanoids clearly plays a significant role in the sensitization of nociceptors to peripheral stimuli, since this effect of bradykinin is reduced by cyclo-oxygenase inhibitors. In vivo, eicosanoids and a variety of other substances stimulate nociceptor activity cooperatively with bradykinin. Evidence that bradykinin is physiologically important as a mediator of pain and inflammation comes from the finding that competitive antagonists at bradykinin receptors show anti-nociceptive and anti-inflammatory activity in animal models.[15]

In sensory neurones bradykinin acts through a membrane receptor to activate membrane enzymes such as phospholipase C (PLC) and phospholipase A_2 (PLA_2)[16], thereby producing various second messengers. Exactly how these are linked to excitation of the neurones remains uncertain. In one proposed sequence of events (*see* Fig. 1) receptor-coupled activation of PLC stimulates production of inositol trisphosphate (IP_3) and diacylglycerol (DAG). IP_3 stimulates calcium mobilization from the endoplasmic reticulum while DAG activates protein kinase C, which in turn opens a cation channel in the neuronal membrane to depolarize and activate the nerve.[17,18] Direct activation of a cation channel by a receptor-linked G-protein is a possibility that cannot be excluded at present. Bradykinin also stimulates the production of arachidonic acid and prostanoids in sensory neurones; this may result directly from activation of PLA_2, or indirectly as a consequence of DAG formation. Weinreich[19] showed the prostaglandins suppress a slow spike after-hyperpolarization in rabbit nodose ganglion cells (Fig. 1), thereby increasing their firing frequency, an effect which could explain the sensitization that these agents induce. The inhibition of the potassium current is mediated via cAMP activation and can also be produced by forskolin, an activator of adenylate cyclase.

The effects of bradykinin in different tissues are mediated via specific receptors of which two subtypes (B_1 and B_2) are well characterized.[20] B_2 receptors predominate in most tissues, and appear to be responsible for nociceptor excitation.[15] Some of the newly-developed B_2-receptor antagonists may prove to be useful clinically in the control of inflammatory pain.

Histamine

Histamine released from mast cells can evoke a variety of responses including antidromic vasodilation, neurogenic plasma extravasation and reactive hyperemia. One stimulus for histamine release is substance P released from peripheral nerve terminals, which interacts with mast cell receptors to induce degranulation. The liberated histamine produces vasodilatation and also interacts with sensory nerve endings. In some experimental situations, high concentrations of histamine have been reported to cause pain, but histamine usually elicits only the sensation of itch.

Eicosanoids

A number of substances derived from the metabolism of arachidonic acid are termed eicosanoids. Notable amongst these are prostaglandins, products of cyclooxygenase enzyme activity, in particular prostaglandin E_2, D_2 and I_2, which are released from a variety of tissues during inflammation. Prostanoids do not generally activate nociceptors directly, but sensitize them to other stimuli and to chemicals, such as bradykinin, present in inflammatory exudates (*see above*). This sensitizing action of prostanoids may be important for the development of peripheral hyperalgesia. Other mechanisms of eicosanoid sensitization may also operate. For example repetitive administration of prostaglandin E_2 to the rat hindpaw produces a prolonged state of hyperalgesia which is partially dependent on *de novo* protein synthesis but, unlike the effect of prostaglandin E_2 on potassium channels, cannot be mimicked by the repeated administration of dibutyryl cyclic AMP.[21]

Leukotrienes and hydroxy-acids

Lipoxygenase products of arachidonic acid metabolism have been shown to play a role in nociceptor sensitization, although the precise mechanisms are poorly understood. Leukotrienes produced during tissue inflammation can act on a variety of cell types but little is known about their effects on sensory neurones. The available information suggests that they act indirectly on sensory neurones by stimulating other cells to release neuroactive agents. In inflamed or damaged tissue, leukotriene D_4 (LTD_4) produces rapid alterations in gene expression in cells such as macrophages and basophils which stimulates an increased synthesis and release of eicosanoids.[22] Furthermore, LTD_4 has been shown to release substance P[23] although it is not certain that the neuropeptide originates from sensory neurones.

LTB_4 has been suggested to play a role in hyperalgesia. This substance, like other leukotrienes, does not act directly on sensory neurons, but is thought to exert an effect through the release of a bioactive hydroxy-acid, (8R, 15S)-diHETE (dihydroxyeicosatetraenoic acid), from polymorphonuclear leukocytes.[24] It is unclear how the liberated diHETE acts on sensory neurones, although a related hydroperoxy-acid increases the excitability of non-mammalian sensory neurones by inhibiting the activity of a K^+ channel.[25] Another possible mode of action is eicosanoid-induced activation of a protein kinase, which is consistent with the observation that the persistent hyperalgesia found after repetitive injections of another hydroxyacid (15-HETE) can be attenuated by an inhibitor of protein kinase C.[26]

Cytokines

Phagocytotic and antigen presenting cells of the immune system release a number of cytokines (interleukins, tumour necrosis factor, interferons) that are important inflammatory agents. These molecules also interact with peripheral nerves, probably by indirect routes that involve mediators produced by other cell types. Interleukin 1β (I1–1β) provides the best evidence for an interaction between cytokines and sensory neurones. Injection of I1–1β in the periphery produces a delayed hyperalgesia that can be antagonisted by α-melanocyte stimulating hormone and tripeptides related to Lys-D-Pro-Thr. These antagonists are antinociceptive in various animal models of inflammatory hyperalgesia.[26,27] One suggestion is that I1–1 activates eicosanoid metabolism in cells such as fibroblasts and causes the release of prostaglandins[27] although the importance of cyclo-oxygenase products in I1–1 induced hyperalgesia has been challenged.[28]

DIRECT ACTIVATORS

Capsaicin–an exogenous activator

Capsaicin (8-methyl-N-vanillyl-6-nonenamide) is a well known algogenic compound found in hot red peppers.[29] It has highly selective effects on mammalian polymodal nociceptors and warm thermoceptors. Local application of capsaicin to skin and mucous membranes activates primary afferent C-neurones to produce a brief burning pain and a longer lasting hyperalgesia.

The rapid and intense activation of nociceptors by capsaicin is due to an underlying membrane depolarization that has been studied in sensory neurones and fibres in vitro. Capsaicin opens a membrane ion channel that is permeable to cations, notably sodium and calcium ions.[30] The current generated by the influx of these ions depolarizes the neurone to the threshold for action potential initiation. The influx of calcium evoked by capsaicin raises the intracellular calcium level in the neurones, which in turn inhibits the voltage dependent calcium conductance[31] which is believed to trigger the events that lead to neurotransmitter release. This inhibitory action of capsaicin on voltage gated calcium currents and transmitter release may therefore be relevant to the acute antinociceptive and anti-inflammatory effects of capsaicin.

The membrane ion channel activated by capsaicin is not obviously one of the known ligand gated or voltage operated channels that exist in neurones. Capsaicin-induced activation of C-neurones is specific to mammalian sensory neurones and is likely to be produced by a direct interaction between capsaicin and a specific membrane receptor. Indirect evidence for this has been provided by studies of the structure-activity relationships of capsaicin derivatives[32–34] including the ultrapotent analogue, resiniferotoxin.[35,36] The presence of a capsaicin receptor has been recently confirmed by the discovery of a competitive antagonist, capsazepine.[37] Capsaicin can also initiate changes in second messenger levels (cGMP, DAG, IP_3 turnover, arachidonic acid release) in sensory neurones.[38,39] These events do not appear to be primary consequences of capsaicin receptor activation, but are probably secondary events triggered by the entry of calcium ions through the activated ion channels.

Exposure to high concentrations of capsaicin blocks conduction in C-fibres and may produce a selective sensory neurotoxicity. This neurotoxicity results from two distinct mechanisms both linked to the agonist actions of capsaicin: osmotic lysis brought about by net accumulation of sodium chloride in the neurone and enzyme mediated damage triggered by the rise in intracellular calcium.[36,40] The neurotoxic actions of capsaicin are unlikely to underlie the antinociceptive and anti-inflammatory effects that last only a few hours and show the characteristics of functional changes without degeneration. Other, more subtle, mechanisms probably mediate these effects of capsaicin.

INTERACTIONS OF C-FIBRES WITH OTHER CELLS

Neurogenic inflammation

It is clear that nociceptive neurons have complex interactions with other cells types that are of critical importance in inflammation and hyperalgesia. A variety of agents generated by tissue damage and by inflammatory cells can either activate or sensitize these nerves. In turn many cells express receptors for neuropeptides, such as substance P, that are released from the peripheral nerve terminals. Substance P induces many of the events associated with neurogenic inflammation; it evokes changes in vascular calibre and permeability that are potentiated by amines (histamine, 5-HT) released from mast cells. It also releases a relaxant factor from vascular endothelium, and stimulates the release of a variety of inflammatory mediators including interleukins, tumour necrosis factor and arachidonic acid.[41] Sensitization or activation of the nerve terminals by the released inflammatory mediators is likely to lead to further peptide release so forming a 'positive feedback' circuit between the sensory neurons and the inflammatory cells (*see* Fig. 2 for some of the possible interactions).

Nerve growth factor

One class of molecules that is important for sensory neurons are growth factors. Among these is nerve growth factor (NGF) which is synthesized and liberated from target tissues. Recent evidence has revealed that NGF production is elevated in inflamed tissues.[42] This finding may have important implications for sensory nerve activation as NGF can influence the properties of sensory neurons by regulating the expression of various genes. NGF stimulates the synthesis of substance P, CGRP and the capsaicin receptor in adult sensory neurons[43,44] and may well alter other properties. Elevated levels of NGF may lead to the increased synthesis and release of peptides in vivo, which would be compatible with the finding of elevated substance P content in inflamed tissues.[45] Tissue NGF levels may also be regulated by peptides released from sensory neurons. Substance P can activate macrophages to release Il–1[46], which, in turn, acts on cells such as fibroblasts and Schwann cells to stimulate NGF production.[47] This would form a feedback loop between substance P release and NGF production that may be important for some of the longer term events associated with inflammation and neuronal sensitization.

Adrenergic receptor activation

There is considerable evidence for the involvement of the sympathetic post-ganglionic neurones in the sensitization of nociceptors to produce peripheral hyperalgesia (*see* McMahon, this issue). Earlier reports that sympathetic stimulation or direct application of catecholamines to an experimental neuroma increased firing in small diameter primary afferent fibres led to the suggestion that noradrenaline, released from sympathetic fibres, had a direct action on primary afferent neurones. However, such a scheme appears unlikely to operate since direct administration of high concentrations of noradrenaline to intact peripheral nociceptors did not produce C-fibre activation.[48] Such findings suggest an indirect mechanism of action. One possibility is that sympathetically mediated hyperalgesia is produced by the activation of adrenergic α-receptors on either sympathetic neurones or non-neuronal cells in the vicinity which leads to the release of prostanoids (prostaglandin I_2) that sensitize nociceptors.[49]

CONCLUSIONS

It is clear that there are complex interactions between neuronal and non-neuronal cells in inflammation with the production of a variety of chemical mediators that are important in nociception.

Some directly open membrane channels while others have more indirect actions that involve the generation and action of second messengers that, in turn, can lead either to activation or to sensitization. Within the latter group are the eicosanoids, which are generated and released by a number of cell types in response to a variety of inflammatory agents. The eicosanoids have important general intra- and inter-cellular roles in nociception. In addition to the well known chemical mediators of nociception other molecules such as cytokines and growth factors, which have been studied relatively little, can have long term effects on nociceptor function and may provide novel targets for the development of analgesic drugs.

REFERENCES

1 Burgess PR, Perl ER. Cutaneous mechanoreceptors and nociceptors. In: Iggo A. ed. Handbook of sensory physiology. Berlin: Springer, 1973: pp. 30–78
2 Besson JM, Chaouch A. Peripheral and spinal mechanisms of nociception. Physiol Rev 1987; 67: 67–186
3 Campbell JN, Raja SN, Cohen RH, Manning DC, Khan AA, Meyer RA. Peripheral neural mechanisms of nociception. In: Wall PD, Melzack R, eds. Pain, 2nd Ed. Edinburgh: Churchill Livingstone, 1989: pp. 22–45
4 Krishtal OA, Pidoplichko VI. A receptor for proton in the nerve cell membrane. Neuroscience 1980; 5: 2325–2327
5 Bevan S, Yeats J. Protons activate a cation conductance in a sub-population of rat dorsal root ganglion neurones. J Physiol 1991; 433: 145–161
6 Krishtal OA, Marchenko SM, Obukhov AG. Cationic channels activated by extracellular ATP in rat sensory neurons. Neuroscience 1988; 27: 995–1000
7 Bean BP. ATP-activated channels in rat and bullfrog sensory neurons: concentration dependence and kinetics. J Neurosci 1990; 10: 1–10
8 Richardson BP, Engel G, Donatsch D, Stadler PA. Identification of serotonin M-receptor subtypes and their specific blockade by a new class of drugs. Nature 1985; 316: 126–131
9 Eschalier A, Kayser V, Gilbaud G. Influence of specific $5HT_3$ antagonists on carageenan-induced hyperalgesia in the rat. Pain 1989; 36: 249–255
10 Boeckaert J, Sebben M, Dumuis A. Pharmacological characterization of 5-hydroxytryptamine$_4$ ($5\text{-}HT_4$) receptors postively coupled to adenylate cyclase in adult guinea pig hippocampal membranes: effect of substituted benzamide derivatives. Mol Pharmacol 1990; 37: 408–411
11 Peters JA, Lambert JJ. Electrophysiology of $5\text{-}HT_3$ receptors in neural cell lines. Trends Pharmacol Sci 1989; 10: 172–175
12 Robertson B, Bevan S. Properties of 5-hydroxytryptamine$_3$ receptor gated currents in adult rat dorsal root ganglion neurones. Br J Pharmacol 1991; 102: 272–276
13 Dunlap K, Fischbach GD. Neurotransmitters decrease the calcium conductance activated by depolarization of embryonic chick sensory neurones. J Physiol 1981; 317: 519–535
14 Christian EP, Taylor GE, Weinreich D (1989) Serotonin increases excitability of rabbit C-fiber neurons by two distinct mechanisms. J Appl Physiol 67; 584–591
15 Steranka LR, Manning DC, DeHaas CJ et al. Bradykinin as a pain mediator:

receptors are localized to sensory neurons and antagonists have analgesic actions. Proc Natl Acad Sci USA 1988; 85: 3245–3249

16 Gammon CM, Allen AC, Morell P. Bradykinin stimulates phosphoinositide hydrolysis and mobilization of arachidonic acid in dorsal root ganglion neurons. J Neurochem 1989; 53: 95–101

17 Burgess GM, Mullaney I, McNeill M, Dunn P, Rang HP. Second messengers involved in the action of bradykinin on cultured sensory neurons. J Neurosci 1989; 9: 3314–3325

18 Thayer SA, Perney TM, Miller RJ. Regulation of calcium homeostasis in sensory neurons by bradykinin. J Neurosci 1988; 8: 4089–4097

19 Weinreich D. Bradykinin inhibits a slow spike after-hyperpolarization in visceral sensory neurons. Eur J Pharmacol 1986; 132: 61–63

20 Regoli D, Barabe J. Pharnaology of bradykinin and related kinins. Pharmacol Rev 1980; 32: 1–46

21 Ferreira SH, Lorenzetti BB, De Campos DI. Induction, blockade and restoration of a persistent hypersensitive state. Pain 1990; 42: 365–371

22 Crook ST, Mattern M, Sarau HM, et al. The signal tranduction system of the leukotriene D_4 receptor. Trends Pharmacol Sci 1989; 10: 103–107

23 Bloomquist EI, Kream RM. Leukotriene D_4 acts in part to contract guinea pig ileum smooth muscle by releasing substance P. J Pharmacol Exp Ther 1987; 240: 523–528

24 Levine JD, Lam D, Taiwo YO, Donatoni P, Goetzl EJ. Hyperalgesic properties of 15-lipoxygenase products of arachidonic acid. Proc Natl Acad Sci USA 1986; 83: 5331–5334

25 Piomelli D, Greengard P. Lipoxygenase metabolites of arachidonic acid in neuronal transmembrane signalling. Trends Pharmacol Sci 1990; 11: 367–373

26 Follenfant RL, Nakamura-Craig M, Garland LG. Sustained hyperalgesia in rats evoked by 15-hydroperoxyeicosatetraenoic acid is attenuated by the protein kinase inhibitor H-7. Br J Pharmacol 1990; 99; 289

27 Ferriera SH, Lorenzetti BB, Bristow AF, Poole S. Interleukin-1β as a potent hyperalgesic agent anatgonized by a tripeptide analogue. Nature 1988; 334: 698–700

28 Follenfant RL, Nakamura-Craig M, Henderson B, Higgs GA. Inhibition by neuropeptides of interleukin-1β-induced, prostaglandin-independent hyperalgesia. Br J Pharmacol 1989; 98: 41–43

29 Bevan S, Szolcsanyi J. Sensory neuron-specific actions of capsaicin: mechanisms and applications. Trends Pharmacol Sci 1990; 11: 330–333

30 Wood JN, Winter J, James IF, Rang HP, Yeats J, Bevan SJ.Capsaicin-induced ion fluxes in dorsal root ganglion cells in culture. J Neurosci 1988; 8: 3208–3220

31 Docherty RJ, Robertson B, Bevan S. Capsaicin causes prolonged inhibition of voltage-dependent calcium currents in adult rat dorsal root ganglion neurones in culture. Neurosci 1991; 40: 513–521

32 Hayes AG, Oxford A, Renolds M, Skingle AH, Smith C, Tyers MB. The effects of a series of capsaicin analogues on nociception and body temperature. Life Sci 1984; 34: 1241–1248

33 Szolcsanyi J, Jancso-Gabor A. Sensory effects of capsaicin congenors. I. Relationship between chemical structure and pain producing potency of pungent agents. Arzneim Forsch Drug Res 1975; 25: 1877–1881

34 James IF, Walpole SJ, Hixon J, Wood JN, Wrigglesworth R. Long lasting agonist activity produced by a capsaicin-like photoaffinity probe. Mol Pharmacol 1989; 33: 643–649

35 Szallasi A, Blumberg PM. Resiniferatoxin, a phorbol-related diterpene, acts as an untrapotent analog of capsaicin, the irritant constituent of red pepper. Neuroscience 1989; 30: 515–520

36 Winter J, Dray A, Wood JN, Yeats JC, Bevan S. Cellular mechanism of action

of resiniferatoxin: a potent sensory neuron excitotoxin. Brain Res 1990; 520: 131–140

37 Bevan S, Hothi S, Hughes GA et al. Development of a competitive antagonist for the sensory neurone excitant, capsaicin. Br J Pharmacol 1991 (In press)

38 Burgess GM, Mullaney I, McNeill M, Coote PR, Minhas A, Wood JN. Activation of guanylate cyclase in rat sensory neurons is mediated by calcium influx; possible role of the increase in cGMP. J Neurochem 1989; 53: 1212–1218

39 Wood JN, Coote PR, Minhas A, Mullaney I, McNeill M, Burgess GM. Capsaicin-induced ion fluxes increase cyclic GMP but not cyclic AMP levels in rat sensory neurones in culture. J Neurochem 1989; 53: 1203–1211

40 Marsh SJ, Stansfeld CE, Brown DA, Davey R, McCarthy D. The mechanism of action of capsaicin on sensory C-type neurones and their axons in vitro. Neuroscience 1987; 23: 275–289

41 Lotz, M., JH Vaughan, Carson DA. Effect of neuropeptides on production of inflammatory cytokines by human monocytes. Science 1988; 241: 1218–1221

42 Weskamp G, Otten U. An enzyme-linked immunoassay for nerve growth factor (NGF): a tool for studying regulatory mechanisms involved in NGF production in brain and peripheral tissues. J Neurochem 1987; 48: 1779–1786

43 Lindsay RM, Lockett C, Sternberg J, Winter J. Neuropeptide expression in cultures of adult rat sensory neurons: modulation of substance P and calcitonin gene-related peptide levels. Neuroscience 1989; 33: 53–65

44 Winter J, Forbes CA, Sternberg J, Lindsay RM. Nerve growth factor (NGF) regulates adult rat cultured dorsal root ganglion neuron responses to capsaicin. Neuron 1988; 1: 973–981

45 Marshall KW, Chiu B, Inman RD. Substance P and arthritis: analysis of plasma and synovial fluid levels. Arthritis Rheumatism 1990; 33: 87–90

46 Hartung HP, Toyka K. Activation of macrophages by substance P: induction of oxidative burst and thromboxane release. Eur J Pharmacol 1983; 89: 301–305

47 Lindholm D, Heumann R, Meyer M, Thoenen H. Interleukin-1 regulates synthesis of nerve growth factor in non-neuronal cells of rat sciatic nerve. Nature 1987; 330: 658–659

48 Lang E, Novak A, Reeh PW, Handwerker HO. Chemosensitivity of fine afferents from rat skin in vitro. J Neurophysiol 1990; 63: 887–901

49 Taiwo YO, Levine JD. Characterization of the arachidonic acid metabolites mediating bradykinin and noradrenaline hyperalgesia. Brain Res 1988; 458: 402–406

British Medical Bulletin (1991) Vol. 47, No. 3, pp. 549–560
© The British Council 1991

Mechanisms of acute visceral pain

F Cervero
Department of Physiology, University of Bristol Medical School, Bristol, UK

Acute visceral pain is dull, aching, ill-defined, badly localized and often referred to remote areas of the body. These properties indicate that the representation of internal organs within the CNS is very imprecise. There is evidence for the existence of specific visceral nociceptors in some viscera and for the existence of non-specific receptors in other internal organs. Some visceral receptors are 'silent' in normal viscera but become active following acute injury or inflammation of the internal organ that they innervate. The number of nociceptive afferent fibres in viscera is very small but these few nociceptive afferents can excite many second order neurones in the spinal cord which in turn generate extensive divergence within the CNS, sometimes involving supraspinal loops. Such a divergent input activates several systems—sensory, motor and autonomic—and thus triggers the general reactions that are charactreistic of visceral nociception: a diffuse and referred pain, and prolonged autonomic and motor activity.

Certain kinds of stimulation of internal organs can cause acute visceral pain. These include: contractures and spasms of the smooth muscle of hollow viscera, distension of hollow viscera, traction or torsion of mesenteries, ischaemia, chemical irritation of mucosae and acute inflammatory states. Other forms of internal injury such as cutting or burning of viscera do not evoke pain and certain internal organs, such as the liver or the lungs are insensitive to pain, that is, the sensation of pain cannot be evoked by any form of stimulation of these viscera.

Acute visceral pain is often very intense, vaguely localized, referred to distant regions of the body and accompanied by powerful motor and autonomic reactons, including spasms of the abdominal musculature and increased sympathetic outflow. Some of these reactions can also appear following cutaneous injury but a prominent feature of acute visceral pain is the disproportion between the amount of internal damage and the intensity of the accompanying reactions. For instance, a relatively minor incident, such as the passing of a kidney stone through the ureter is one of the most painful events experienced by humans and is always accompanied by overpowering motor and autonomic reactions.

VISCERAL SENSORY RECEPTORS AND VISCERAL NOCICEPTORS

Internal organs are innervated by one category of peripheral receptor whose stimulation evokes no sensations. Examples of these receptors are the arterial baroreceptors that signal changes in blood pressure, the carotid body chemoreceptors that signal changes in blood gases, the lung inflation and deflation receptors that transmit signals about pulmonary ventilation and the atrial volume receptors whose signals are used for the homeostatic control of body fluids. Since their activation does not lead to the perception of a conscious sensation they cannot be regarded as part of the 'sensory' innervation of viscera but as a component of the 'afferent' innervation of internal organs. The distinction between sensory and afferent innervation of viscera has been discussed previously in some detail[1,2] and highlights a fundamental difference between the mechanisms of cutaneous and visceral sensation.

On the other hand, certain forms of visceral stimulation can evoke pain (see above) which demonstrates the existence of sensory receptors in internal organs capable of being activated by the stimuli that will be perceived as painful. What is still the object of some argument is the encoding mechanism by which visceral afferent signals become sensory messages capable of evoking a conscious perception. There are essentially two different mechanisms for the encoding of visceral nociceptive events:

(i) receptors responsible for the sensations of visceral pain are the same population of visceral receptors responding to innocuous stimuli and responsible for visceral reflex actions. These receptors would respond to noxious stimuli with higher frequencies of firing;

(ii) receptors responsible for the sensations of visceral pain are a different population of visceral receptors which respond to the same stimuli that evoke visceral reflex actions but with different thresholds or by different mechanisms. This view postulates the existence of specific visceral nociceptors.

There is experimental evidence for the existence of both specific nociceptors and nonspecific sensory receptors in the viscera (e.g. see Refs. 3–5). It is possible that both kinds of visceral receptor act in parallel conveying information to the central nervous system about noxious visceral events. Also, it could be that the activation of specific visceral nociceptors results in more restricted and clear-cut forms of visceral pain, whereas the vague and dull forms of internal discomfort are due to general stimulation of non-specific visceral receptors.

Some gastrointestinal sensations, such as those evoked by colorectal distension, begin as non-painful feelings of distension and evolve towards an uncomfortable and painful sensation as the distension progresses. These properties can be paralleled by the electrophysiological properties of some colonic receptors[6] which respond with greater impulse frequencies to colonic distensions of increasing magnitude. On the other hand, viscera such as the gall bladder, the biliary ducts and the ureter, from which pain is the only sensation that can be evoked appear to be innervated by specific visceral nociceptors[7,8] (*see* Fig. 1). In any case, it is a dangerous oversimplification to relate the final perception of a

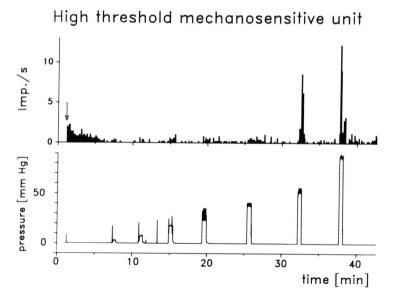

High threshold mechanosensitive unit

Fig. 1 Responses of a high threshold mechanosensitive unit from the guinea-pig's ureter to controlled increases in intraluminal pressure. Probing of the receptive field (arrow) induced long lasting after-discharges. (*Modified from*: Ref. 8).

visceral sensation to the properties of the peripheral sense organ at the origin of the sensory pathway. The final conscious perception of visceral pain depends on the way in which the central nervous system integrates the afferent visceral inflow, regardless of the peripheral encoding mechanism.

Sensitization of visceral nociceptors

One possible trigger for the sensation of visceral pain could be the sensitization of visceral nociceptors. According to this interpretation visceral nociceptors, which normally have a relatively high threshold and respond only to intense forms of stimulation, become abnormally sensitive by decreasing their threshold for activation thus responding to mild forms of stimulation. As a result, reflex activity normally triggered only by a strong stimulus will appear now as a result of the ordinary physiological process of internal homeostasis. This disrupts physiological patterns, evokes abnormal motility and secretion and leads to the perception of visceral pain.

There is considerable experimental evidence in support of the idea of sensitization of visceral nociceptors. For instance, Haupt et al.[6] have shown that sensory receptors in the colon of the cat become spontaneously active as a consequence of ischaemia of the gut. In this study, ischaemia of the colon induced an increased and irregular spontaneous activity in the sensory receptors which became also sensitized to pressure and chemical stimuli.

In a study of the afferent innervation of the ureter, Cervero and Sann[8] have also demonstrated a similar mechanism. They used an in vitro preparation of the guinea-pig ureter with an intact nerve supply and measured the distension thresholds of mechanosensitive afferent fibres with receptive fields in the wall of the ureter. They found that if the ureter was not perfused intraluminally with oxygenated fluid the afferent fibres showed a higher background activity and a lower pressure threshold than in preparations in which the ureters were perfused with oxygenated fluid at a physiological flow rate (Fig. 2). They concluded that an insufficient oxygen supply, reproducing the conditions of in vivo ischaemia, sensitized the high threshold nociceptors in the ureter to a lower threshold and to a greater responsiveness.

'Silent' nociceptors

Over the last few years, a number of experimental studies on the innervation of deep and visceral structures have provided evidence

Thresholds of ureteric afferent fibres

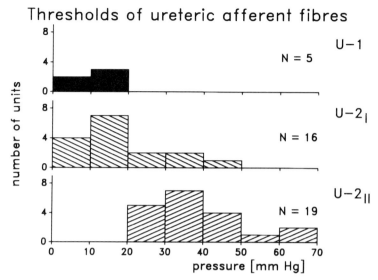

Fig. 2 Distribution of the response thresholds to intraluminal pressure increases of ureteric afferent units. *Top*: low threshold units (U-1); *bottom*: high threshold units (U-2-II); *middle*: U-2 units from experiments in which the mucosa of the ureter was not perfused with oxygenated saline solution (U-2-I). (*From*: Ref 8).

for the existence of sensory receptors that are only activated by persistent damage or inflammation of the tissue that they innervate (*see* Ref. 9). These are believed to be 'silent' nociceptors, normally unresponsive to physiological forms of stimulation but being able to respond to mild stimuli when the tissue suffers persistent damage.

The largest amount of evidence so far for the existence of silent nociceptors comes from studies on the sensory innervation of the joints[10] but this kind of nociceptor has also been found in the colon and urinary bladder.[11] Receptors in the wall of the bladder have been found which could not be activated in the normal state but that became responsive to bladder distension and contraction following the induction of an inflammation of the bladder with turpentine.

PERIPHERAL AND CENTRAL DISTRIBUTION OF VISCERAL AFFERENT FIBRES

It has been known for some time that the total number of primary afferent fibres involved in the transmission of visceral nociceptive information is quite small.[12] This low density of innervation is particularly striking when taking into account the large surface area of the viscera and is probably the reason for the diffuse nature of visceral pain. Recent studies, using neuronal tracing and labelling methods, have established that visceral afferent fibres constitute less than 10% of the total afferent inflow to the thoracolumbar spinal cord.[13] It must be noted that this region of the spinal cord receives its somatic input from the body areas with the poorest sensory discrimination (i.e. the back and the abdomen), whereas the visceral input to the thoraco-lumbar cord mediates pain from all upper abdominal organs including the stomach, the duodenum, the biliary tract, the pancreas and the small intestine. Yet the former sensations require 90% or more of the total afferent input to the spinal cord whereas all visceral pain from the upper abdomen is mediated by less that 10% of all spinal afferents.

Although visceral afferent fibres represent a very small proportion of the total afferent inflow to the spinal cord, it is well known that these few fibres can activate a large number of neurones in the cord through extensive functional divergence.[1,2,4,5] These central actions are expressed as increases in the excitability of somatic and autonomic reflexes occurring in parallel with the unpleasant sensory experience. Thus, the activation of visceral nociceptors evokes persistent increases in muscle tone, changes in viscero-motor and viscero-secretory reflexes and profound cardiovascular alterations as well as a strongly aversive sensation of pain.

It is surprising that these large and generalized effects can be triggered by such a small number of visceral primary afferent fibres. Morphological studies on the mode of termination of visceral afferent fibres within the spinal cord indicate that the widespread effects caused by the activation of visceral nociceptive afferents are not mediated by extensive anatomical divergence of the visceral projection but are probably the consequence of functional divergence of visceral impulses within the spinal cord. The anatomical pattern of termination of visceral afferent fibres within the spinal cord has been examined in sacral, lumbar and thoracic region of the spinal cord in several animal species.[14] Visceral afferent fibres display a consistent pattern of central termination throughout the spinal cord with areas of projection in Laminae I and V but sparing the intermediate dorsal horn (Laminae II, III and IV). Contralateral projections of afferent fibres in the splanchnic nerve have also been described. Visceral afferent fibres reach the dorsal horn via Lissauer's tract and join medial and lateral bundles of fine fibres that run along the edges of the dorsal horn. Fibres from these bundles penetrate the grey matter and terminate within Laminae I and V of the dorsal horn (Fig. 3).

CENTRAL MECHANISMS OF ACUTE VISCERAL PAIN

Dorsal horn and other spinal cord neurones can be classified into two main groups depending on the presence or absence of an excitatory visceral input. Some neurones are not driven by visceral afferent fibres and can only be excited from their somatic receptive fields (somatic neurones). Other cells have, in addition to their somatic input, an excitatory visceral drive (viscero-somatic neurones). Thus, visceral sensations can only be mediated through convergent signals via somatosensory pathways. No evidence has been found for the presence of a sensory pathway exclusively concerned with the transmission of visceral sensory signals. In agreement with the anatomical data on the mode of termination of somatic and visceral afferent fibres within the spinal cord, the locations of somatic and viscerosomatic neurones show a differential distribution within the spinal grey matter. Somatic neurones are mainly located in Laminae II, III and IV of the dorsal horn whereas viscero-somatic cells are located in Lamina I, Lamina V and in the ventral horn. The majority of somatic cells are mechanoreceptive, that is, capable of responding to low intensity mechan-

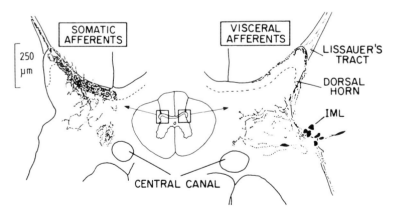

Fig. 3 Reconstruction from 3 (left) and from 7 (right) 80 μm transverse serial sections of the projections of somatic (left) and visceral (right) afferent fibres to the T9 segment of the spinal cord of the cat. Horseradish peroxidase was applied to the intercostal nerve of the T9 spinal segment (left) and to the splanchnic nerve (right). (*Modified from*: Ref. 24).

ical stimulation of the skin but not to noxious stimulation. In contrast, most viscero-somatic cells are driven by somatic nociceptors either exclusively or in addition to their low threshold inputs.[15]

In the lower thoracic spinal cord, about 30% of all viscerosomatic neurones have been found to respond to distension of the gall bladder and of the biliary ducts.[15] All these cells were excited at noxious levels of distension, i.e. levels of biliary pressure which evoked pseudaffective reflexes, including transient changes in blood pressure. Similarly, spinothalamic tract cells in the sacral spinal cord of the monkey can be excited by noxious stimulation of the testicles.[16] Thus, it would appear that for those organs from which the only sensation that can be evoked is that of pain, noxious intensities of stimulation are necessary to excite viscerosomatic neurones in the spinal cord.

A different pattern of activation of spinal cord neurones has been reported using distension of the colon as a visceral stimulus.[17] In this case, several populations of cells could be distinguished depending on their threshold responses to colonic distension and on the adaptation rate of the neuronal discharge. Some of these cells responded to low intensity distensions of the colon and increased their levels of firing at higher, noxious, intensities. Other cells, however, responded only to noxious distension of the large intestine. It is possible that the cells that respond to innocuous stimulation of the colon are not concerned with sensation from this organ but with the regulatory aspects of gastrointestinal function. On the other hand, it is important to realise that non-painful sensations of colorectal distension can be perceived normally and that these sensations can become painful if the distension increases or persists. Therefore, there is a parallel between the neuronal responses described above and the psychophysics of the sensations evoked by colorectal distension.

The observations that visceral afferent fibres converge onto somatosensory spinal cord neurones, that most of these neurones have a somatic nociceptive input, that the visceral input to these cells is also of nociceptive nature, and that some of these viscerosomatic cells project through nociceptive pathways provide strong experimental support for all the main postulates of the 'convergence-projection' theory of referred visceral pain.[18] The referral of the visceral sensation is therefore the consequence of the activation of pathways normally concerned with the integration of somatic nociceptive signals. These pathways will be activated by their visceral inputs with a very different spatial and temporal pattern than that normally generated by their cutaneous drives. In particular, many more cells will be activated by a visceral noxious stimulus and over a greater region of the spinal cord than by somatic stimuli. Because of the large number of cells activated by a visceral noxious stimulus, the sensation is usually felt in a large area of the body whose overall size depends on the intensity of the noxious stimulus.

Central modulation of viscero-somatic neurones

It is known that a volley of impulses arriving in the spinal cord via somatic or visceral afferent fibres inhibits the response of a viscero-somatic neurone to a second volley in any of its peripheral drives.[15] This inhibition, which can last for up to one second, is produced by a neuronal network wholly contained within the spinal cord, as can be shown by the fact that spinalization of the experimental animals does not eliminate these inhibitory effects. Therefore, the activation of spinal viscero-somatic neurones by any of their inputs will produce a subsequent reduction in the excitability of these cells to further afferent impulses.

Examination of the input properties of viscero-somatic neurones, their ascending projections and the nature and strength of their supraspinal control have revealed several categories of viscero-somatic neurone that can be reduced to two very broad groups:[19]

(i) Viscero-somatic neurones with a restricted visceral input and subject to descending inhibitory control. These neurones are a minority among viscero-somatic neurones and are located mainly in the superficial dorsal horn. They are activated by ipsilateral visceral afferent fibres and have restricted somatic receptive fields from which they can only be driven by noxious stimulation of the skin. Neurones in this region of the dorsal horn are known to project to the brain via spino-thalamic pathways and seem to be part of the nociceptive-specific system of the superficial dorsal horn.[20]

These cells are subject to segmental inhibitory controls and to descending inhibition of supraspinal origin.[21,22] They can be inhibited by electrical stimulation in the Nucleus Raphe Magnus (NRM) and it is likely that this inhibition originates from NRM cell bodies. These cells are good candidates for a transmission

Class 2, lamina V

GB=+

■ Initial receptive field

— After gallbladder stimulation

···· During spinal block

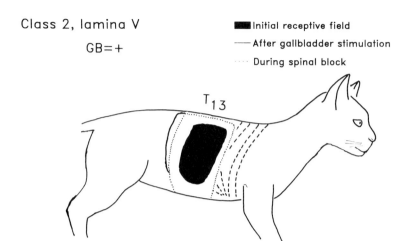

Fig. 4 Changes in the size of the cutaneous receptive field of a viscerosomatic neurone from the thoracic spinal cord of the cat. The black area represents the size of the receptive field prior to any stimulation. This receptive field increased in size to the continuous/dotted border following a 3 minute period of noxious distension applied to the gall bladder. After recovery, spinalization of the animal increased the receptive field size from the black area to the dotted line area. The neurone was Multireceptive (Class 2), was located in Lamina V and could be driven by noxious stimulation of the gall bladder. (*Unpublished work from*: Laird and Cervero).

system that could mediate the more immediate sensory effects resulting from visceral noxious stimulation.

(ii) Viscero-somatic neurones with a diffuse visceral input and subect to descending excitatory and inhibitory control. These are neurones located in the deep dorsal horn and in the ventral horn and driven by bilateral visceral inputs. They are the most numerous group of viscero-somatic neurones, have large and multireceptive somatic receptive fields often involving inputs of deep somatic origin and their visceral inputs are mediated or reinforced by supraspinal loops.[21,22] A proportion of them project to the Reticular Formation of the brain stem and its seems that their descending excitation originates from rostral medullary centres.

These cells have their excitability increased by visceral nociceptive stimulation and remain in a highly excitable state as a consequence of their spinal-bulbo-spinal positive feedback loops. Current work in our laboratory (Laird & Cervero unpublished) has shown that the cutaneous receptive fields of viscero-somatic neurones in the thoracic spinal cord of the cat can increase in size following noxious stimulation of the visceral input to the cells (Fig. 4). This increase persists for some time after the stimulation and can also be expressed by reversible spinalization of the experimental animals, a procedure known to release tonic descending inhibition on spinal cells. It is therefore conceivable that these cells could be concerned with the processing of signals that lead to the cutaneous hyperalgesia and the persistent increases in motor and autonomic reflex activity that are so characteristic of acute visceral pain.

Taking into account these experimental observations on the spinal and supraspinal integration of visceral sensory systems, a model can be proposed that addresses the way in which visceral nociceptive signals, including those of visceral origin are processed. In this model, the perception of visceral pain is the consequence of the activation of a sensory channel driven by somatic and visceral inputs. The final perception depends on the interaction between the incoming excitation from viscera and the segmental and supraspinal inhibitory systems triggered by other peripheral inputs. In addition, descending excitatory systems are responsible for the presence of sustained activity within the system that may be expressed as enhanced motor and autonomic reflexes or as persistent pain (*see* Refs. 4 and 23 for further details).

REFERENCES

1 Cervero F. Mechanisms of visceral pain. In: Lipton S and Miles J eds. Persistent Pain Vol. IV, London: Grune & Stratton, 1983: pp. 1–19

2 Cervero F. Visceral nociception: peripheral and central aspects of visceral nociceptive systems. Philos Trans R Soc 1985: 308; 325–337

3 Jänig W, Morrison JFB. Functional properties of spinal visceral afferents supplying abdominal and pelvic organs with special emphasis on visceral nociception. In: Cervero F, Morrison JFB, eds. Visceral Sensation. Progr Brain Res Amsterdam: Elsevier, 1986, Volume 67, pp 87–114

4 Cervero F. Visceral Pain. Proceedings of the Vth World Congress on Pain. Pain Res & Clin Manag 1988; 3: 216–226

5 Cervero F, Foreman RD. Sensory innervation of the viscera. In: Loewy AD, Spyer KM, eds. Central regulation of autonomic functions. New York: Oxford University Press, 1990; pp. 104–125

6 Haupt P, Jänig W, Kohler W. Response pattern of visceral afferent fibres, supplying the colon, upon chemical and mechanical stimuli. Pflügers Archiv 1983; 398: 41–47

7 Cervero F. Afferent activity evoked by natural stimulation of the biliary system in the ferret. Pain 1982; 13: 137–151

8 Cervero F, Sann H. Mechanically evoked responses of afferent fibres innervating the guinea-pig's ureter: an in vitro study. J Physiol 1989; 412: 245—266

9 McMahon SB, Koltzenburg M. Novel classes of nociceptors: beyond Sherrington. Trends Neurosci 1990; 13: 199–201

10 Schaible HG, Schmidt RF. Effects of an experimental arthritis on the sensory properties of fine articular afferent units. J Neurophysiol 1985; 54: 1109–1122

11 Häbler HJ, Jänig W, Koltzenburg M. Activation of unmyelinated afferent fibres by mechanical stimuli and inflammation of the urinary bladder in the cat. J Physiol 1990: 425; 545–562

12 Procacci P. A survey of modern concepts of pain. In: Vinken PJ, Bruyn GW eds. Handbook of Clinical Neurology. Vol. I. Amsterdam: Elsevier, 1969: pp. 114–146

13 Cervero F, Connell LA, Lawson SN. Somatic and visceral primary afferents in the lower thoracic dorsal root ganglia of the cat. J Comp Neurol 1984; 228: 422–431

14 De Groat WC. Spinal cord projections and neuropeptides in visceral afferent neurones. In Cervero F, Morrison JFB. eds., Visceral Sensation. Progr Brain Res Amsterdam: Elsevier, 1986, Volume 67, pp 165–187

15 Cervero F, Tattersall JEH. Somatic and visceral sensory integration in the thoracic spinal cord. In: Cervero F., Morrison JFB, eds. Visceral Sensation. Progr Brain Res Amsterdam: Elsevier, 1986, Volume 67, pp 189–205

16 Milne RJ, Foreman RD, Giesler jr GJ, Willis WD. Convergence of cutaneous and pelvic visceral nociceptive inputs onto primate spinothalamic neurones. Pain 1987; 11: 163–183

17 Ness TJ, Gebhart GF. Characterization of neuronal responses to noxious visceral and somatocutaneous stimuli in the medial lumbrosacral spinal cord of the rat. J Neurophysiol 1987; 57: 1867–1892

18 Ruch TC. Visceral sensation and referred pain. In Fulton JF. ed. Howell's Textbook of Physiology, 15th edn. Saunders: Philadelphia, 1946: pp. 385–401

19 Cervero F, Lumb BM. Bilateral inputs and supraspinal control of viscerosomatic neurones in the lower thoracic spinal cord of the cat. J Physiol 1988; 403: 221–237

20 Cervero F, Tattersall JEH. Somatic and visceral inputs to the thoracic spinal cord of the cat: Marginal Zone (Lamina I) of the dorsal horn. J Physiol 1987; 388: 383–395

21 Tattersall JEH, Cervero F, Lumb BM. Effects of reversible spinalization on the visceral input to viscero- somatic neurones in the lower thoracic spinal cord of the cat. J Neurophysiol 1986; 56: 785–796

22 Tattersall JEH, Cervero F, Lumb BM. Viscero- somatic neurones in the lower thoracic spinal cord of the cat: excitations and inhibitions evoked by splanchnic and somatic nerve volleys and by stimulation of brain stem nuclei. J Neurophysiol 1986; 56: 1411–1423

23 Cervero F. Neurophysiology of Gastrointestinal Pain. Clin Gastroenterol 198; 2: 183–199

24 Cervero F, Connell LA. Distribution of somatic and visceral primary afferent fibres within the thoracic spinal cord of the cat. J Comp Neurol 1984; 230: 88–98

British Medical Bulletin (1991) Vol. 47, No. 3, pp. 561–583
© The British Council 1991

Clinical management of acute pain

D M Justins
Pain Management Centre, St Thomas' Hospital, London, UK

P H Richardson
Department of Academic Psychiatry, United Medical and Dental School, St Thomas' Hospital, London, UK

The clinical management of acute pain has been impeded by traditions and misconceptions which have resulted in suboptimal application to the patient of the currently available methods of pain control. The search for new drugs and exotic ways to deliver them has further obscured many of the basic principles which should guide management. Standard regimens fail because of the wide, unpredictable variability in pain intensity, patient characteristics, and pharmacological responses. Treatment needs to be individualized for each patient. Unrelieved acute pain produces psychological, physiological and socioeconomic consequences. Pre-emptive analgesia may damp down the development of both immediate and long-term pain following surgery and adequate psychological preparation can improve coping abilities. The delivery of opioid analgesics can be improved using patient controlled analgesia or spinal administration in some cases. Regional analgesia, often using simple techniques, can produce excellent pain relief. Overall management and staff education should be delegated to an acute pain service.

This chapter will deal mainly with postoperative pain but the methods of pain relief can be applied with equal benefit to any form of acute pain such as: obstetrics, intensive care, trauma, burns and other medical and surgical conditions—including acute pancreatitis, myocardial infarction, sickle disease, peripheral vascular occlusion, ureteric colic, orthopaedics, osteomyelitis, gout, prolapsed intervertebral disc, cancer, pathological fracture and raised intracranial pressure.

The aetiology of acute pain is usually obvious and is linked to a site of ongoing nociceptive stimulation. Unlike most chronic pain, the expectation of patient and staff is that the pain will be of relatively short duration and that it will resolve completely.

Current management

Many reports suggest that acute pain is often very poorly managed with 30 to 70% of patients reporting inadequate analgesia after conventional treatment although staff frequently believe that analgesia is adequate.[1,2] Medical and nursing staff seem reluctant to use the maximum ordered analgesia both in respect of dosage and frequency of administration. Children fare particularly badly. Often no analgesia at all is ordered, or if ordered it is either not given or a weaker drug substituted in preference to an opioid. The various surveys reveal some surprising staff attitudes. Only 20% of staff aim to achieve complete pain relief; drugs are chosen randomly with little regard for the nature and severity of the pain; and patients who complain too much are criticized for having a 'low pain threshold'.

The literature is overflowing with reports of new drugs, new techniques, and the cyclical rediscovery of old methods. Can this be justified? Does good pain control reduce morbidity and mortality?

BENEFITS OF CONTROLLING ACUTE PAIN

'There is nothing the body suffers the mind may not profit by'
George Meredith

Despite earlier attitudes the psychological, physiological, and socioeconomic effects of unrelieved acute pain are considerable.

Psychological

Unrelieved acute pain causes distress, suffering, and sleep deprivation which leads to falling morale and rising anxiety.

Physiological

Respiratory: Pain impairs breathing and coughing and predisposes the patient to respiratory complications. Effective analgesia counters these effects and makes physiotherapy easier. *Cardiovascular*: Hypertension and tachycardia produced in response to pain may be harmful to a patient with cardiac disease and the increase in cerebral blood flow may be dangerous for a head injury patient. *Gastrointestinal* motility is impaired. *Mobility* is restricted by pain, and pressure sores develop. *Thromboembolism* is more likely. The *endocrine-metabolic response* is only partly mediated by pain and even total pain relief with epidural bupivacaine and morphine plus systemic indomethacin has only a slight effect following upper abdominal operations.[3] There are pronounced physiological benefits to mother and child in relieving the pain of labour.

Socioeconomic

Convalescence is slower and hospital stay longer after poor pain control. Increased nursing attention is required. Consumer satisfaction is reduced and patients face future medical intervention with trepidation.

PROBLEMS OF CONTROLLING ACUTE PAIN

The biggest problem in acute pain management is the unpredictable variability of pain (incidence, intensity and time course), of patient characteristics and of pharmacological factors.

Pain intensity varies widely between patients even after similar operations. Individual assessment is essential. Various factors affect the incidence and intensity.

Factors beyond control

The most important factor is the site of the operation. Thoracic or upper abdominal operations usually produce severe pain of at least 2 to 3 days duration. Drain sites, a urinary catheter or a nasogastric tube can also be painful. Age, sex, race, and social background exert variable influences on the pain experience.[4] Personality, anxiety trait, neuroticism, extroversion and the placebo response[5] may influence pain. The significance of the pain and past pain experiences are important.

Factors within control

The operative technique and skin incision can greatly influence pain. Cutting diathermy may be kinder than the knife.[6] Other factors include ward design, comfort, sleep, distractions, and psychological aspects such as anxiety state and feelings of fear or helplessness. Important pharmacological influences are the choice and dose of drug, and the practical aspects of delivery such as route, mode and frequency. There is very widespread variation in individual responses to treatment and in analgesic requirements. One critical factor which can be controlled is the attitude of the medical staff, particularly that of the nurses.

There is considerable variation in onset, pattern and duration of post operative pain. The onset time is influenced by such things as premedication and perioperative drugs. The pattern may be constant, cyclical (e.g. colic), or incident (e.g. related to coughing). Pain intensity usually declines with time. The widespread variation in the intensity and time course of postoperative pain creates a dilemma when pre-emptive analgesia is provided because some patients will receive unnecessary treatment. The measurement and assessment of acute pain is difficult and depends upon subjective reports.

PSYCHOLOGICAL ASPECTS OF ACUTE PAIN

There is now extensive evidence that a variety of psychological factors may influence the experience of pain as well as pain related cognitions and behaviour. These include—mood, personality, attention and other perceptual processes, expectations and the placebo response, reinforcement contingencies, observational learning, various social and ethnocultural factors, the therapist–patient relationship, predictability and perceived control of the painful stimulus, and anxiety.[7] Whilst a few of these factors have been documented more extensively in the field of chronic pain (e.g. reinforcement contingencies in relation to learned pain behaviour) the majority have been studied in relation to both acute and chronic pain.

The status of the available evidence linking psychological factors with experienced pain is variable. For example whilst the placebo effect has been widely recorded in laboratory and clinical research on pain, the specific psychological processes associated with its occurrence (e.g. classical conditioning, cognitive dissonance, anxiety reduction etc) remain unclear.[8] Moreover, whilst anxiety is frequently regarded as an important influence on pain, the available clinical evidence concerning the nature of the relationship between pain and anxiety is far from clearcut.[9] As Craig (1989) has pointed out, much of this evidence raises unanswered questions about the direction of causality. Moreover the measures used to assess both pain and anxiety are often confounded[10] adding conceptual confusion to the empirical uncertainty.

The most frequently noted psychological consequence of acute pain appears to be anxiety. However, depression, irritability, sleep problems, interpersonal withdrawal, increased sensitivity to external stimuli, delirium and even acute psychotic reactions have also been recorded.[11]

Consistent with the diversity of psychological influences on pain has been the development of a wealth of different psychologically-based therapies including—autogenic and muscular relaxation, hypnosis, stress inoculation and anxiety management methods, systematic desensitization, biofeedback, individual and group psychotherapy, cognitive coping strategies training, goal setting and graded activity scheduling, and contingency management procedures.[12]

Studies of the psychological management of acute clinical pain can be divided into two major categories: firstly, those concerned with pain as a consequence of illness or injury (e.g. studies of burns pain); and secondly those of pain which may arise as a direct consequence of medical or dental procedures (e.g. surgery, cardiac catheterization).

In contrast with the vast body of published work on chronic pain management[13] relatively few studies have systematically evaluated the benefits of psychological management of non-iatrogenic acute clinical pain. Moreover, from the research which has been conducted firm conclusions are limited by a series of methodological shortcomings (e.g. small sample sizes, poor measurement).[14] A notable exception is the work on burned patients. In this area there is now a promising body of evidence from well controlled studies that cognitive and behavioural methods (including relaxation, hypnosis and stress management) can promote reductions in both pain and pain-related distress.[14]

The psychological management of pain associated with stressful medical procedures has been widely investigated. The majority of studies have examined the effects of different forms of psychological preparation on patients' responses during potentially painful procedures or in the recovery period following surgery. Early work linking preoperative anxiety and distress with postoperative recovery[15] gave rise to the suggestions that appropriate preparation could ameliorate the recovery process in a number of ways. Subsequent research has gone some way towards identifying which particular preparatory procedures (e.g. information provision, relaxation instructions) affect which particular outcomes (e.g. pain, distress, analgesic consumption) through what mechanisms of action (e.g. anxiety reduction, altered expectations, improving coping skills).

Four principal categories of preparatory procedure have been identified.[16]

1. *Information provision*—including details of the procedures to be undergone by the patient both during and after the intervention, as well as sensory information preparing the patient for sensations, such as pain or nausea.

2. *Behavioural instructions*—in the form of training to relax, to cough properly or to use a trapeze to turn over in bed.

3. *Cognitive methods*—encouraging patients to think more positively about their experiences and avoid 'catastrophizing'. Cognitive methods may also include instruction in techniques (e.g. somatisation, imaginative transformation) designed to alter the perception of pain.

4. *Psychotherapeutic approaches*—exploring patients' emotional responses, either individually or in groups.

The use of these methods is predicted upon differing hypotheses concerning their role in reducing pain and distress. Information provision could promote more realistic expectations in the patient and reduce anticipatory anxiety. Relaxation exercises might be expected to reduce pain through attention diversion or by lowering muscle tension at the site of the wound. As well as any direct physical effects, instructional preparation may also increase patients' sense of personal control over painful or distressing stimuli. Cognitive methods should improve overall coping skills. Psychotherapeutic procedures may be expected to reduce emotional distress.

The above methods have been used with adults and children during preparatory interviews conducted by surgeons, anaesthetists, nurses and psychologists, and using videotaped models. Numerous outcome measures have been employed, including various kinds of subjective pain rating as well as records of analgesic consumption. Weinman and Johnston[17] have recently reviewed evidence from controlled trials for the effectiveness of these preparatory methods. Overall the findings indicate that all methods are capable of reducing analgesic consumption, albeit by potentially different pathways of action. Where subjective pain ratings are concerned the results are mixed. Relaxation and cognitive methods have generally produced encouraging results. The other methods have not yet established their usefulness.

In view of their additional beneficial effects upon other modalities of patient response (e.g. mood, duration of postoperative stay[17]) and the ease with which they can be incorporated into normal care, there is much to be said for the routine introduction of psychological methods of preparation for all potentially painful or stressful medical procedures. However further research is needed into the precise nature of their influence before their full therapeutic potential can be exploited.

FAILURE TO RELIEVE ACUTE PAIN

The complexities and unpredictable variability of pain and pain control partially explain the failure of postoperative analgesia in many patients but pain control fails most frequently because medical staff ignore this variability and fail to use available methods to full potential. The responsibility for acute pain care is often disjointed with no clear guidelines.

Doctors fail because of ignorance, inexperience, tradition, and overwork. The more senior they become the less they are concerned with pain control. Anaesthetists are often confined to operating theatres but they have the knowledge and skills which are needed to deal with the various problems.

The nurses (particularly the ward sisters) are the key distributors of analgesia but they also fail because of ignorance, inexperience, tradition and overwork. Unfounded fears of addiction and respiratory depression deter them from using opioids. Controlled drug regulations impede them further. The nurse's attitudes and beliefs may hinder rational treatment.

Patients too may contribute by failing to ask for, or expect, adequate pain relief.

PREVENTION OF PAIN

Analgesic premedication or nerve blocks peformed before surgery commences may reduce the incidence of postoperative pain (preemptive analgesia) by damping down peripheral and dorsal horn sensory mechanisms. The idea that prevention is better than cure is not original!

The combination of opioid premedication and peroperative neural blockade leads to an apparently reduced incidence of postoperative pain.[18] Surgery performed with the use of local or spinal anaesthesia may be less painful postoperatively.[19] The benefit from a nerve block performed at the time of operation can last for at least 4 days; long after any local anaesthetic blockade has disappeared. Nonsteroidal anti-inflamatory drugs (NSAID) such as piroxicam[20] or diclofenac[21] preoperatively reduce postoperative analgesic needs.

The provision of good perioperative analgesia may influence long term sequelae and minimise persistent postsurgical pain syndromes.[22] Epidural analgesia for three days prior to amputation may help to eliminate post-amputation pain syndromes.[23]

Kehlet's group reported that pain could be totally eliminated in virtually all patients using a balanced technique of low dose extradural bupivacaine plus morphine, and systemic piroxicam after surgery performed under combined intrathecal, epidural and general anaesthesia.[24] Balanced analgesia follows balanced anaesthesia.

OBJECTIVES OF PAIN MANAGEMENT

The aims of management in acute pain are to minimize discomfort, facilitate recovery, and avoid treatment side effects. Any method must be effective, safe, feasible, and cost effective and should balance analgesia and side effects on one hand against pain and the patient's wishes on the other.

METHODS OF ACUTE PAIN MANAGEMENT

1. *Prevention*—Psychoprophylaxis, pre-emptive analgesia
2. *Remove cause*—Surgery, radiotherapy, splinting
3. *Inhibit peripheral response to acute injury*—NSAIDs, ice packs
4. *Interrupt peripheral transmission*—Neural blockade, cryoanalgesia
5. *Alter spinal processing*—Spinal opioids and other drugs, stimulation techniques
6. *Alter central processing*—Opioids, other analgesics, psychotropic drugs
7. *Psychological methods*—Stress reduction, coping strategies, information.

OPIOIDS IN ACUTE PAIN MANAGEMENT

The prescription of a potent opioid is the most common method of postoperative analgesia yet pain control is often inadequate because medical staff ignore pharmacological influences. The most obvious influences apart from choice of drug are route, mode, time and frequency of administration. The individual response to treatment also varies because of pharmacokinetic and pharmacodynamic differences.

Pharmacokinetics describes the uptake, distribution and elimination of the drug and there is wide variation between individuals, and sometimes in the same individual at different times. Following intramuscular injection peak concentration, time to peak concentration, and the duration of effective blood concentration may vary by at least a factor of five.[25] Nonparental routes are subject to even greater variability in absorption.

The patient characteristics which may influence analgesic pharmacokinetic variability include: age (the elderly have a diminished volume of distribution), hepatic disease, renal disease, acid base balance, hypothermia, hypothyroidism and concurrent drug administration.

Even if all the pharmacokinetic variables are overcome so that a constant plasma opioid concentration is maintained, individual patients will still experience varying degrees of pain relief. The concentration at which each patient becomes pain free also varies by a factor of 3 or 4 and has been described as the Minimum Effective Analgesic Concentration. The validity of this has been challenged.[26]

Standard regimens cannot cater for this variability and analgesic administration must be individualized for each patient. The ideal is a steady plasma concentration that will maintain analgesia without causing toxicity. As concentration increases so does the incidence of side effects. The route of administration is one of the most important determinants of success.

Available routes for opioid administration

Intramuscular

Simplicity and economy are the only advantages. The injections are painful and there is wide variation in absorption, onset, peak, duration, toxicity so that 'on demand' administration is unsatisfactory. Peak concentration rises with subsequent injections and this route does not avoid the risk of opioid respiratory depression.[27] Regular administration can produce high quality analgesia. Patient controlled administration has been used but requires larger doses than with intravenous injection. A slow release intramuscular preparation is available.

Subcutaneous

This is a simple and often effective method, particularly as an infusion, although it is prone to wide variability because of unpredictable uptake from the subcutaneous tissue.

Oral

The oral route is not ideal for acute pain control because first pass metabolism by the liver results in variable bioavailability and leads to unpredictable results. Postoperative gastric stasis, vomiting and inability to swallow also limit the usefulness of this route. Controlled release preparations have been used satisfactorily in some postoperative situations, but not in others.

Sublingual

This route avoids the problems of first pass metabolism and inability to swallow. Sublingual buprenorphine has been used with some success although it is less potent than morphine and has a slow onset time so that the drug is not ideal for severe acute pain. Side effects such as nausea vomiting and sedation are common.

Buccal

Morphine was not superior to placebo in a trial reported by Manara et al.

Inhaled

A pilot study with inhaled fentanyl suggests that it is an effective method of analgesia which merits further investigation.[29]

Rectal

New sustained release preparations[30] may overcome problems of variable absorption and uneven control: a useful route in children.

Transdermal

Fentanyl patches have produced significant analgesia in postoperative pain.[31] Uptake and distribution is slow so precise control is difficult but this offers apparent simplicity with minimal staff demands and may be useful when resources are limited.

Intravenous

This route offers the advantage of immediate, reliable uptake of drug by the systemic circulation producing rapid onset so that the dose can be titrated for each patient. The main disadvantage is the narrow safety margin between adequate analgesia and serious side effects so that most intravenous techniques demand a high level of supervision and special equipment such as syringe pumps.

Modes of intravenous delivery

Intermittent bolus has the advantage of rapid predictable onset allowing titration of dose against pain but toxicity is common and the duration of analgesia is brief resulting in a pattern of peaks and troughs for pain control. This method is labour intensive if used for long periods but is suitable for acute perioperative administration. Regular intermittent administration is the basis of most PCA (Patient Controlled Analgesia).

Continuous infusion avoids the peaks and troughs of intermittent administration and allows smoother pain control but infusion pharmacokinetics are complex, especially initially. Most authors suggest an initial pain relieving bolus dose prior to infusion but this dose bears little relationship to the maintainance dose rate subsequently needed to control pain. Acute tolerance may develop during infusions.[32] The safety margin is narrow and high levels of nursing surveillance are essential as the concentration rises slowly over a long period.[33] In most cases the patient has little control over the infusion. Intravenous infusions have proved to be very useful in infants and children, and even for neonates after major surgery.

Combined continuous infusion plus intermittent bolus on-demand will in theory allow control of background pain and acute exacerbations whilst avoiding continual high blood concentration.

Patient Controlled Analgesia (PCA)

Medical staff generally control analgesic administration but pain is a subjective experience and it is only the patient who knows the exact pain intensity at any one time. With PCA a machine will administer a preset dose of drug when the patient presses a button. The machine contains a microprocessor which will prevent misuse or overdose. Some machines also provide a background infusion which can be altered in response to the number of demands made by the patient.

The feeling of autonomy is a potent influence on morale and confidence. Rapid onset of analgesia is possible; dose can be titrated against pain giving the ability to cope with fluctuating pains without the need to maintain constant maximal effective plasma concentration; and nursing time for pain control can be reduced. Patient control avoids compulsory analgesia for the patient who does not need it.

PCA use requires motivation and understanding from the patient. The system is pain contingent so uneven control may result and no demands can be made during sleep. The patient may feel isolated and mobility is restricted. The equipment is expensive but simple devices are available.[34]

PCA machines have also been used for intramuscular, subcutaneous, and epidural administration, although the complex kinetics of these routes render them less than ideal.

PCA prescription

PCA prescription should stipulate: drug, concentration, loading dose, demand dose, rate of administration, lock-out interval, maximum dose over 4 hours, and any concurrent mandatory infusion. Poorly prescribed PCA (dose too large or too small, or lockout too long) may lead to inadequate analgesia or a high incidence of side effects.[35] The relationship between the demand dose and lockout interval, and the optimal infusion profile for each dose are still being determined.

Evaluation of PCA

There is a high degree of patient acceptance in most reports.[36] Success (efficacy and absence of side effects) is not inevitable and depends mostly on the size of the demand dose. If the bolus dose is too small then a large proportion of patients fail to achieve adequate analgesia.[35] It is claimed that patients tend to maintain relatively constant plasma concentration. Side effects, particularly nausea and vomiting, may occur in a significant proportion of patients.

Is PCA better

Is PCA better than other methods? Although some trials compare optimally conducted PCA with a poor alternative, many studies suggest that PCA is superior to conventional intramuscular injections.[37] Other claimed advantages include reductions in hospital stay, nursing time, and costs but some studies are critical. Zacharias et al. concluded that a properly supervised continuous infusion is as good as PCA.[38]

Drug consumption

Drug consumption during PCA varies widely but overall dosage is usually reduced. Morphine consumption over 24 hours may vary from 5.2 to 164.0 mg and shows an inverse correlation with age but no correlation with weight, height or body surface area.[4]

Safety

Respiratory depression is the major concern but most reports suggest that it is not common in practice if reasonable doses are used. Respiratory depression is more common with a background infusion; a morphine dose greater than 2 mg; and with pre-existing respiratory problems or a low respiratory rate.[35,36] Equipment problems, such as self triggering or deprogramming, are unusual.

Concurrent infusion

There are conflicting opinions about whether a background infusion improves the quality of pain relief. Patients with infusions use much larger analgesic doses and run an increased risk of respiratory depression.[36,39] A variable rate infusion can be altered in response to the demand frequency.

Indications

PCA is suitable for anyone capable of understanding the concept and pressing a button. More specific indications include respiratory disease, obesity, the elderly, and some children.

Contraindications

Failure to understand, inability to press the button, or inadequate supervision.

The practicalities of using PCA have been detailed by Notcutt.[36] The issues include: education, equipment, logistics, preoperative preparation, supervision, protocols, monitoring, and audit.

SPINAL OPIOIDS

Epidural and intrathecal opioid administration has gained widespread and often uncritical acceptance in many centres. The theoretical advantage of pure segmental analgesia without motor, sympathetic, or sensory blockade, or central depression has been superseded by a more complex reality. Morgan (1989) has reviewed the subject and concludes that there is no evidence that spinal opioids provide analgesia superior to that produced with other routes of administration although they certainly produce more prolonged analgesia at much smaller doses.[40] Other authors do claim superior analgesia with spinal administration.[41] Studies have demonstrated that patients receiving this form of analgesia experience reduced mortality and morbidity and spend less time in hospital.[42–44]

Clinical experience reveals a wide variation in response (and consequently in recommended doses) and this is probably a reflection of among other things the very complex pharmacokinetics of epidural opioids.[45] Most of an epidural dose is taken up by the systemic circulation and not the dorsal horn as was first suggested. Many different drugs have been used. Morphine is the most popular but more lipid soluble drugs may have advantages.

Intrathecal injection produces prolonged analgesia but continuous techniques are less popular and the incidence of side effects is higher in some reports.[46] A small dose of diamorphine added to intrathecal bupivacaine can produce prolonged analgesia.[47] Epidural catheters are much more familiar although the resulting analgesia may be less predictable but many claim that infusions result in better analgesia and fewer side effects.[48] PCA systems may allow lower drug dosage.[49]

These techniques possess all the procedural risks of spinal injections and also a high incidence of inherant side effects. Respiratory depression is the most worrying of these complications and a number of predisposing factors have been suggested including age, posture, prolonged surgery, concommitant opioid or sedative administration, and the dose, volume, and lipophilicity of the drug. Poorly fat soluble, hydrophilic drugs such as morphine remain in the CSF for a prolonged period, thus producing the prolonged analgesia but also increasing the risk of respiratory depression following cephalad spread.

Nausea and vomiting, urinary retention, ileus, pruritis and sedation occur with often unacceptably high frequency in many reports. Sedation is especially important for it may be a more reliable indicator of impending respiratory depression than even respiratory rate. Prophylactic transdermal scopolamine patches reduce nausea in patients receiving epidural morphine.[50]

These techniques are not safe in a general ward unless close monitoring is provided for up to 24 hours after the final administration of spinal opioid. Naloxone must be instantly available. No systemic opioids or other CNS depressants should be given during the period of spinal opiate analgesia.

Spinal opioids are not the answer to all acute pain problems but can be very useful in selected cases, such as after major thoracoabdominal surgery.

Spinally administered nonopioid drugs such as ketamine, somatostatin, clonidine, calcitonin, baclofen, and midazolam are unlikely to find widespread use in acute pain at the moment.

NEWER OPIOIDS

Buprenorphine, pentazocine, nalbuphine, butorphanol and meptazinol are synthetic partial agonists or mixed agonist-antagonists which have a weaker analgesic action than morphine. Respiratory depression is less of a problem but the weaker analgesia and troublesome side effects such as nausea, vomiting, and dysphoria, limit the use of these drugs in acute pain management.

NONOPIOID ANALGESICS

NSAIDs are especially useful in pain caused by inflammation and in bone pain but produce a high incidence of side effects—including gastric ulceration, abnormal blood clotting and renal disturbance. Drugs such as ketorolac[51], and diclofenac[21] can be given by injection. Pioxicam given preoperatively reduces postoperative analgesic requirements.[20] Prophylactic intravenous infusion of indomethacin can improve postoperative pain management in children.[52] These newer drugs may play an increasing role in postoperative analgesia particularly after the first day when used in combination with other methods.[24] In our hospital we have been investigating regional intravenous salicylate injection for orthopaedic pain.

Ketamine has marked analgesic activity and a subcutaneous infusion of morphine and ketamine at low dose provides reliable analgesia. Steroids will reduce postoperative pain, particularly after oral surgery.[53] An intravenous infusion of low dose lignocaine decreases the severity of postoperative pain and is devoid of side effects.[54] Nitrous oxide and oxygen mixture (Entonox) is useful in acute pain but bone marrow toxicity and worries about pollution limit long term application. Anxiolytics potentiate opioid analgesia and may become more important with perhaps patient controlled anxiolysis in the future.

REGIONAL ANALGESIA

Regional analgesic techniques (nerve blocks) simply aim to interrupt nociceptive transmission in the peripheral nervous system and are capable of producing complete pain relief (including incident pain) without any central depressant effect on consciousness or respiration. Reduced muscle tone and sympathetic block may enhance healing. Central blocks may suppress the stress response and improve respiration. Neural blockade may actually suppress the spinal cord changes which potentiate pain and predispose to persistent painful sequelae. As well as reducing pain, regional techniques used for surgery may reduce the impact of the postoperative fatigue syndrome.[55]

Unfortunately there are disadvantages as well. Acute pains may involve both somatic and visceral pathways that represent a wide spread of spinal segments which may not be easily blocked. The performance of some blocks requires a high degree of skill and is time consuming. Failures occur even in the best hands. Factors other than precision of needle placement influence outcome (drug, dose, volume, spread, vascularity). The drugs only act for a limited time and repeated administration may be impractical. Side effects are also significant and include immediate complications, such as needle trauma or local anaesthetic toxicity, and delayed effects resulting from motor or autonomic blockade. Tachyphylaxis can limit effectiveness. Some cases require increased supervision.

Methods of regional analgesia

Regional blocks require meticulous attention to detail. One of the greatest dangers lies in exceeding the dose limits of the local anaesthetic and thus causing toxicity. Neural damage may occur if the needle traumatises the nerve of an anaesthetised patient.

Topical and wound infiltration

Regional techniques do not have to be complex and topical application of local anaesthetic as a spray, ointment, or local infiltration at the time of operation, or wound perfusion afterwards are very simple and often remarkably effective. The benefits may last for at least 24 hours.[56] Topical lignocaine is effective following circumcision. Intra-articular infusion is effective following menisectomy.

Nerve blocks

Blocks such as digital, wrist, ankle, intercostal, ilioinguinal, penile, and femoral are simple to perform and are very useful especially in paediatric and outpatient surgery. Intercostal blocks produce very effective analgesia following unilateral abdominal incisions and reduce the incidence of postoperative pulmonary complications but the risk of pneumothorax is a major disadvantage.[57] Single rib, large volume injections may be just as effective as multiple levels injections.

Plexus block

A catheter can be inserted near the brachial[58] or lumbar plexus[59] and an infusion of local anaesthetic used to provide continuous analgesia following limb surgery.

Intrapleural block

Local anaesthetic is infused via a catheter inserted into the intrapleural space and very effective analgesia has been produced following thoracotomy and unilateral abdominal operations but potential side effects are a major disadvantage.[60]

Paravertebral blocks

Paravertebral blocks will relieve pain[61] but spread of solution is variable and unpredictable, and the risk of pneumothorax is significant.

Epidural analgesia

Epidural analgesia displays all the advantages and disadvantages of regional analgesia in postoperative pain control. These blocks can provide complete pain relief; improve respiratory function; suppress the endocrine-metabolic response; reduce the incidence of thromboembolic episodes; improve gastrointestinal function; and speed recovery. The reverse side of the coin reveals a high incidence of significant side effects such as hypotension, urinary retention, and muscular weakness.

The lumbar and thoracic routes are most commonly used but caudal injections can provide excellent pain relief in adults and children following many urological, pelvic, or perineal operations. Epidural injections can abolish pain so that it need no longer be an inevitable accompaniment of childbirth.

Recommended techniques use either intermittent top-ups or a continuous infusion of either local anaesthetic alone, or a mixture of dilute local anaesthetic and opioid. The use of a mixture allows a smaller dose of both opioid and local anaesthetic to be used and produces superior analgesia.[62] A key point is to site the catheter tip at the centre of the required band of analgesia.

An intrathecal catheter (e.g. 28 guage) using very small doses has been recommended for the elderly patient with a fractured femur.

Cryoanalgesia

Cryoanalgesia has been used to produce very prolonged analgesia, most particularly after thoracotomy when the surgeon can apply the cryoprobe to the intercostal nerves under direct vision, but it does not block visceral pain and the prolonged numbness may worry the patient. Gough et al.[63] found cryoanalgesia inferior to epidural fentanyl infusion.

STIMULATION INDUCED ANALGESIA

Transcutaneous electrical nerve stimulation [TENS] has not been shown to be universally effective.[64] Electroacupuncture given immediately after surgery reduced opioid requirements in the first 2 hours[65] but there is little evidence to support acupuncture as an effective remedy.

SELECTION OF MANAGEMENT

Choice of the most appropriate method will be governed by: (1) the nature of the surgery; (2) the intensity and expected duration of the pain; (3) the availability of drugs and expertise; (4) the efficacy and side effects of the available methods; and (5) patient factors such as preexisting illness, age and psychological state. Combination techniques, for example using a local anaesthetic block, a nonsteroidal anti-inflammatory drug and an opioid may provide better analgesia with fewer side effects than reliance upon a single method.

Special problems in postoperative pain management may arise in paediatric and geriatric practice, following day-case surgery, and in patients with severe respiratory disease, obesity, head injury, or drug addiction.

SAFETY AND MONITORING

Fear of complications has been one of the main impediments to improving acute pain management. These fears are often unfounded although respiratory depression can follow opioid administration by any route but is a particular risk during spinal or intravenous administration.[27] Respiratory rate does not correlate with hypercapnia.[66]

The provision of adequate monitoring and nursing surveillence is essential when techniques such as PCA, intravenous infusion and spinal analgesia are in use. Some patients may be nursed on a High Dependancy Unit. This will be suitable for those with preexisting illness or those having very major surgery which is likely to cause severe pain. The majority of patients will have to be nursed on general wards where monitoring, such as pulse oximetry, is unlikely to be widely available. It is necessary to establish a standard protocol which describes: (1) routine monitoring of respiratory rate, sedation, other side effects, pain score, and drug consumption (acceptable limits must be well defined); (2) immediate management schemes for any complication or problem; and (3) immediately available help.

ACHIEVING IMPROVEMENTS

Improved management of acute pain can be achieved by the rational application of existing drugs and methods. This requires changes in orientation and attitude of doctors and nurses as well as the provision of special equipment and dedicated nursing areas. Education must be aimed at patients as well as staff. A positive step is the formation of an Acute Pain Service which may include anaesthetist, nurse, psychologist, physiotherapist and pharmacist.[67] This is the multidisciplinary approach which has worked so well in chronic pain now applied to acute pain. The acute pain service should be responsible for the day to day management of acute pain, the training of medical and nursing staff, audit, and research.

REFERENCES

1 Kuhn S, Cooke K, Collins M, Jone JM, Mucklow JC. Perceptions of pain relief after surgery. Br Med J 1990; 300: 1687–1690
2 Owen H, McMillan V, Rogowski D. Postoperative pain therapy: a survey of patients' expectations and their expeiences. Pain 1990; 41: 303–307
3 Kehlet H. Surgical stress: the role of pain and analgesia. Br J Anaesth 1989; 63: 189–195
4 Burns JW, Hodsman NBA, McLintock TTC, Gillies GWA, Kenny GNC, McArdle CS. The influence of patient characteristics on the requirement for postoperative analgesia. Anaesthesia 1989; 44: 2–6
5 Hashish I, Hai HK, Harvey W, Feinmann C, Harris M. Reduction of postoperative pain and swelling by ultrasound treatment: a placebo effect. Pain 1988; 33: 303–311
6 Hussain SA, Hussain S. Incisions with knife or diathermy and postoperative pain. Br J Surg 1988; 75: 1179–1180
7 Pearce SA. Chronic pain: A biobehavioural perspective In: Christie MJ, Mellett PG, eds. The Psychosomatic Approach: Contemporary Practice of whole-person care. London: Wiley, 1986: pp. 217–237
8 Richardson PH. Placebos: their effectiveness and modes of action In: Broome A, ed. Health psychology: Processes and applications. London: Chapman and Hall, 1989: pp. 34–56
9 Craig KD. Emotional Aspects of Pain. In: Wall PD, Melzack R, eds. Textbook of Pain, 2nd edn, Edinburgh: Churchill Livingstone, 1989: pp. 220–230
10 Gross RT, Collins FL. On the relationship between anxiety and pain: a methodological confounding. Clin Psychol Rev 1981; 1: 375–386
11 Cousins M. Acute and Postoperative Pain. In: Wall PD, Melzack, eds. Textbook of Pain. 2nd edn. Edinburgh: Churchill Livingstone, 1989; pp. 285–305
12 Melzack R. Psychological Aspects of Pain In: Cousins MJ, Bridenbough PO,

eds. Neural blockade in clinical anaesthesia and management of pain. 2nd edn. Lippincott: Philadelphia, 1988: pp. 845–860

13 Pearce SA, Richardson PH. Chronic Pain: Treatment. In: Lindsay S, Powell G, eds. A handbook of clinical adult psychology. Aldershot: Gower, 1987: pp. 579–594

14 Choinere M. The treatment of burns. In: Wall PD, Melzack R, eds. Textbook of pain. 3rd edn. Edinburgh: Churchill Livingstone, 1989: pp. 402–407

15 Janis IL. Stress and frustration. New York: Harcourt Brace Johanovich, 1971

16 Johnston M. Counselling and psychological methods with postoperative pain: a brief review. Health psychology update 1990; 5: 8–14

17 Weinman J, Johnson M. Stressful medical procedures: an analysis of the effects of psychological interventions and of the stressfulness of the procedures. In: Maes S, Defares P, Sarason IG, Spielberger CD, eds. Proceedings of the First International Expert Conference on Health Psychology, London: Wiley, 1989

18 McQuay HJ, Carroll D, Moore RA. Postoperative orthopaedic pain—the effect of opiate premedication and local anaesthetic blocks. Pain 1988; 33: 291–295

19 Tverskoy M, Cozacov C, Ayache M, Bradley EL, Kissen I. Postoperative pain after inguinal herniorrhaphy with different types of anaesthesia. Anesth Analg 1990; 70: 29–35

20 Hutchison GL, Crofts SL, Gray IG. Preoperative piroxicam for postoperative analgesia in dental surgery. Br J Anaesth 1990; 65: 500–503

21 Campbell WI, Kendrick R, Patteson C. Intravenous diclofenac sodium. Does its administration before operation suppress postoperative pain? Anaesthesia 1990; 45: 764–766

22 Cousins MJ. Acute pain and the injury response: immediate and prolonged effects. Regional Anesthesia 1989; 14: 162–179

23 Bach S, Noreng MF, Tjellden NU. Phantom limb pain in amputees during the first 12 months following limb amputation after preoperative lumbar epidural blockade. Pain 1988; 33: 297–301

24 Dahl JB, Rosenberg J, Dirkes WE, Mogensen T, Kehlet H. Prevention of postoperative pain by balanced analgesia. Br J Anaesth 1990; 64: (in press)

25 Austin KL, Stapleton JV, Mather LE. Multiple intramuscular injections: a major source of variability in analgesic responses to meperidine. Pain 1980; 8: 47–62

26 Owen H, Kluger MT, Plummer JL. Variable of patient controlled analgesia 4: the relevance of bolus dose size to supplement a background infusion. Anaesthesia 1990; 45: 619–622

27 Wheatley RG, Sommerville ID, Sapsford DJ, Jones JG. Postoperative hypoxaemia: comparison of extradural, i.m. and patient-controlled opioid analgesia. Br J Anaesth 1990; 64: 267–275

28 Manara AR, Bodenham AR, Park GR. Analgesic efficacy of perioperative buccal morphine. Br J Anaesth 1990; 64: 551–555

29 Worsley MH, Macleod AD, Brodie MJ, Asbury AJ, Clark C. Inhaled fentanyl as a method of analgesia. Anaesthesia 1990; 45: 449–451

30 Hanning CD, Vickers AP, Smith G, Graham NB, McNeil ME. The morphine hydrogel suppository: a new sustained release rectal preparation. Br J Anaesth 1988; 61: 221–228

31 Rowbotham DJ, Wyld R, Peacock JE, Duthie DJR, Nimmo WS. Transdermal fentanyl for the relief of pain after upper abdominal surgery. Br J Anaesth 1989; 63: 56–59

32 Marshall H, Porteous C, McMillan I, MacPherson SG, Nimmo WS. Relief of pain by infusion of morphine after operation: does tolerance develop? Br Med J 1985; 291: 19–21

33 Catling JA, Pinto DM, Jordan C, Jones JF. Respiratory effects of analgesia after cholecystectomy: comparison of continuous and intermittent papaveretum. Br Med J 1980; 2: 478–480

34 Rowbotham DJ, Wyld R, Nimmo WS. A disposable device for patient-controlled analgesia with fentanyl. Anaesthesia 1989; 44: 922–924

35 Owen H, Plummer JL, Armstrong I, Mather LE, Cousins MJ. Variables of patient controlled analgesia. Bolus size. Anaesthesia 1989; 44: 7–10

36 Nottcutt WG, Morgan RJM. Introducing patient-controlled analgesia for postoperative pain control into a district general hospital. Anaesthesia 1990; 45: 401–406

37 Tamsen A. Comparison of patient controlled analgesia with constant infusion and intermittent intramuscular regimens. In: Harmer M, Rosen M, Vickers MD, eds. Patient controlled analgesia. London: Blackwells, 1985: pp. 111–123

38 Zacharias M, Pfeifer MV, Herbison P. Comparison of two methods of intravenous administration of morphine for postoperative pain relief. Anaesth Intensive Care 1990; 18: 205–209

39 Owen H, Szekeley SM, Plummer JL, Cushnie JM, Mather LE. Variables of patient controlled analgesia. Concurrent infusion. Anaesthesia 1989; 44: 11–13

40 Morgan M. The rational use of intrathecal and extradural opioids. Br J Anaesth 1989; 63: 165–188

41 Yeager MP, Glass DD, Neff RK, Brinck-Johnsen T. Epidural anesthesia and analgesia in high risk surgical patients. Anesthesiology 1987; 66: 729–736

42 Stenkamp SJ, Easterling TR, Chadwick HS. Effect of epidural and intrathecal morphine on the length of hospital stay after cesarian section. Anesth Analg 1989; 68: 66–69

43 Cullen ML, Staren ED, El Ganzouri A, Logas WG, Ivankovitch AD, Economov SG. Continuous epidural infusion for analgesia after major abdominal operations: a randomised, prospective, double blind study. Surgery 1985; 98: 718–726

44 Loper KA, Ready LB, Nessly M, Rapp SE. Epidural morphine provides greater pain relief than patient-controlled intravenous morphine following cholecystectomy. Anesth Analg 1989; 69: 826–828

45 Nordberg G, Hansdottir V, Kvist L, Mellstrand T, Hedner T. Pharmacokinetics of different epidural sites of morphine administration. Eur J Clin Pharmacol 1987; 33: 499–504

46 Stoelting RK. Intrathecal morphine—an underused combination for postoperative pain management. Anesth Analg 1989; 68: 707–709

47 Reay BA, Semple AJ, Macrae WA, MacKenzie N, Grant IS. Low dose intrathecal diamorphine analgesia following major orthopaedic surgery. Br J Anaesth 1989; 62: 248–252

48 Lee A, Simpson D, Whitfield, Scott DB. Postoperative analgesia by continuous extradural infusion of bupivacaine and diamorphine. Br J Anaesth 1988; 60: 845–850

49 Marlowe S, Engstrom R, White PF. Epidural patient controlled analgesia (PCA): an alternative to continuous epidural infusions. Pain 1989; 37: 97–101

50 Loper KA, Ready LB, Dorman BH. Prophylactic transdermal scopolamine patches reduce nausea in postoperative patients receiving epidural morphine. Anesth Analg 1989; 68: 144–146

51 Power I, Noble DW, Douglas E, Spence AA. Comparison of i.m. ketorolac trometamol and morphine sulphate for pain relief after cholecystectomy. Br J Anaesth 1990; 65: 448–455

52 Maunuksela E-L, Olkkola KT, Korpela R. Does prophylactic intravenous infusion of indomethacin improve the management of postoperative pain in children. Can Anaesth Soc J 1988; 35: 123–127

53 Korman B, McKay RJ. Steroids and postoperative analgesia. Anaesth Intensive Care 1985; 13: 395–398

54 Cassuto J, Wallin G, Hogstrom S, Faxen A, Rimback G. Inhibition of postoperative pain by continuous low dose intravenous infusion of lidocaine. Anesth Analg 1985; 64: 971–974

55 Kehlet H. Anesthetic technique and surgical convalescence. Acta Chir Scand 1988; (Suppl 550): 182–191

56 Partridge BL, Stabile BE. The effect of incisional bupivacaine on postoperative narcotic requirements, oxygen saturation and length of stay in the post-anaesthesia care unit. Acta Anaesth Scand 1990; 34: 486–491

57 Sabanathan S, Mearns AJ. Efficacy of continuous extrapleural intercostal nerve block on post-thoracotomy pain and pulmonary mechanics. Br J Surg 1990; 77: 221–226

58 Sarma VJ. Long-term continuous axillary plexus blockade using 0.25% bupivacaine. Acta Anaesth Scand 1990; 34: 511–513

59 Anker-Moller E, Spangsberg N, Dahl JB, Christensen EF, Schultz P, Carlsson P. Continuous blockade of the lumbar plexus after knee surgery: a comparison of the plasma concentrations and analgesic effect of bupivacaine 0.250% and 0.125%. Acta Anaesth Scand 1990; 34: 468–472

60 Strombskag KE, Minor B, Steen PA. Side effects and complications related to intrapleural analgesia: an update. Acta Anaesth Scand 1990; 34: 473–477

61 extradural infusions of bupivacaine for pain relief after thoracotomy. Br J Anaesth 1989; 62: 204–205

62 Scott NB, Morgensen T, Bigler D, Lund C, Kehlet H. Continuous thoricic extradural 0.5% bupivacaine with or without morphine: effect on quality of blockade, lung function and the surgical stress response. Br J Anaesth 1989; 62: 253–257

63 Gough JD, Williams AB, Vaughan RS, Khalil JF, Butchart EG. The control of post-thoracotomy pain. A comparative evaluation of thoracic epidural fentanyl infusions and cryoanalgesia. Anaesthesia 1988; 43: 780–783

64 McCallum MID, Glynn CJ, Moore RA, Lammer P, Phillips AM. Transcutaneous electrical nerve stimulation in the management of acute postoperative pain. Br J Anaesth 1988; 61: 308–312

65 Christensen PA, Noreng M, Andersen PE, Nielsen JW. Electroacupuncture and postoperative pain. Br J Anaesth 1989; 62: 258–262

66 Holley FO, Van Steennis C. Postoperative analgesia with fentanyl: pharmacokinetics and pharmacodynamics of constant rate i.v. and transdermal delivery. Br J Anaesth 1988; 60: 608–613

67 Ready LB, Oden R, Chadwick HS et al. Development of an anesthesiology-based post-operative pain management service. Anesthesiology 1988; 68: 100–106

British Medical Bulletin (1991) Vol. 47, No. 3, pp. 584–600
© The British Council 1991

Mechanisms of sympathetic pain

S B McMahon
Department of Physiology, St Thomas' Hospital Medical School, United Medical and Dental Schools, London, UK

In some chronic pain states, notably causalgia and reflex sympathetic dystrophy, activity in sympathetic efferent neurones can exacerbate the pain and sympathectomies relieve it. These patients are said to have sympathetically maintained pain (SMP). In normal tissue, activity in postganglionic sympathetic efferents does not produce pain, nor is it capable of activating nociceptive sensory neurones. It can, however, induce modest firing in some mechanoreceptors.

SMP is often held to result from a vicious circle of events which include changes in peripheral and central somatosensory processes, and most importantly a positive feedback element in the form of sympathetic efferent neurones which, by activating sensory neurones in the periphery, completes the vicious circle. Several specific hypotheses have been advanced as to the primary pathophysiological cause of pain in these patients. Suggestions, largely deriving from observations on animal models, include: ephaptic transmission, adrenergic receptors on sensory neurones, indirect coupling of sympathetic and sensory neurones, sensitization of nociceptive afferents, and, in the central nervous system, sensitization of dorsal horn neurones. All these suggestions have some supporting evidence, but none are able to adequately explain all the disturbances seen in patients with SMP.

This chapter will consider to what extent and by what mechanisms the sympathetic nervous system may contribute to the abnormal sensory experiences of several types of chronic pain patient. The most important conditions are those of causalgia and reflex sympathetic dystrophy. Causalgia is a condition that occasionally follows trauma to a major nerve. The term was coined by Mitchell in the middle of the last century[1] to indicate the presence of persistent burning pain in such cases. The more general term reflex sympathetic dystrophy is used to categorize patients with some or all of the following symptoms: spontaneous burning pain; hyperalgesia (used here to indicate both pain to normally innocuous events and increased sensitivity to noxious events); hyperpathia (delayed and exaggerated painful response to stimuli[2]); disturbances of vasomotor and sudomotor control; dystrophic changes in the peripheral tissues such as abnormalities of hair and nail growth and osteoporosis. Whilst there is still much confusion in the use of these terms, reflex sympathetic dystrophy is generally used when the condition is not associated with obvious peripheral nerve trauma. Precipitating events include minor tissue trauma and fractures, non-traumatic nerve lesions such as those seen in diabetes, and even lesions to the central nervous system. The term algodystrophy is sometimes used instead of reflex sympathetic dystrophy, as is Sudeck's atrophy, although strictly this refers to a radiological finding.[3]

There are two main reasons for believing that the sympathetic nervous system may be important in the genesis of pain in these conditions. Firstly, sympathetic function is frequently abnormal. The skin of the affected region is often initially warm and red and later pale and cold. Anhydrosis or hyperhydrosis may be present. The dystrophic changes that occur are likely to be secondary to changes in blood flow to the area.[4] The second, and more compelling, reason for implicating the sympathetic nervous system is that manoeuvres which alter sympathetic activity frequently alter the patient's pain. For instance, visual and auditory stimuli, emotional disturbance or thermal stress all provoke sympathetic arousal and can all exacerbate the pain in these patients.[5,6] Similarly, iontophoresis of adrenergic agents into the affected territory can induce pain.[7] Conversely, surgical or chemical sympathectomy sometimes produce a rapid and complete relief of the spontaneous pain and hyperalgesia (*see* Charlton, this issue). However, not all patients show improvement with sympathetic blockade. This has given rise to the idea that some patients have sympathetically maintained pain (SMP) and others sympathetically independent pain (SIP).[8] Some other observations support this distinction. It is a clinical impression that the presence of hyperpathia is a positive indicator of the likely benefits of sympathectomy[9] and Raja et al.[10] have reported that patients with SMP are more likely to have a hyperalgesia to cold stimuli. On the other hand, the definition of SMP is entirely pragmatic, depending on the outcome of regional blocks. Since some authors maintain that a long series of blocks is sometimes necessary to produce pain relief (some patients have had more than 30[11]), this obviously creates a practical problem in the diagnosis of SIP.

SYMPATHETIC EFFECTS IN HEALTHY TISSUE

If we accept that in several pathophysiological states sympathetic efferents can produce pain and hyperalgesia, an obvious question is to what extent similar effects can occur in normal healthy tissue. We know that many peripheral targets, in addition to blood vessels, receive a sympathetic supply. For instance, there is good evidence for an innervation of muscle spindles, Pacinian corpuscles and other specialized end-organs in skin.[12] We might also expect a modification of sensory inflow to occur secondary to changes in blood flow or piloerection. It is therefore not surprising that physiological experiments have identified some actions of sympathetic efferent in normal skin. Cold thermoreceptors can be excited by low frequency stimulation of the sympathetic trunk.[13] Similarly, some sensitive mechanoreceptors with unmyelinated axons are also transiently excited[14,15] an effect which is probably due to small changes in the tension in the tissues secondary to vasomotor changes. Sensitive mechanoreceptors with large diameter axons have also been examined. Most workers have found that hair follicle afferents are partially desensitized by sympathetic stimulation, with a time course that makes it unlikely to be a consequence of altered blood flow.[15,16] However, in skin yielding good piloerection, Roberts & Foglesong[17] have found that hair follicle afferents can be excited by sympathetic stimulation. Some slowly adapting mechanoreceptors can also be activated.[17,18]

A most important question, of course, is whether nociceptors are excited by sympathetic stimulation. Here all workers agree that for normal nociceptors, both with Aδ or C axons, no direct excitation occurs.[14,15,19-21] Together, these studies suggest that in normal tissue sympathetic activity will have only modest sensory effects. It is therefore no surprise that sympathetic activation or intradermal injections of noradrenaline do not lead to pain or hyperalgesia in man or animals.[7,22] Sympathectomy also does not lead to a permanent alteration of pain sensitivity.[23]

THEORIES OF SYMPATHETICALLY MEDIATED PAIN

Any theory seeking to explain the mechanism of SMP needs to address several issues derived from clinical experience. Firstly, it must, of course, explain exactly how sympathetic activity modulates pain. The effectiveness of sympathetic blockade produced by regional guanethidine treatment implies that there is a peripheral interaction between sympathetic efferents and sensory afferents, and there are several suggestions as to the nature of this interaction (see below). Secondly, it is not yet clear which afferent fibre types are responsible for signalling the pain and hyperalgesia. The fact that regional anaesthesia usually relieves the condition suggests that some afferent activity is responsible. We might intuitively suspect that the most likely explanation would be the presence of aberrant activity in nociceptors. However, clinical observations are not clear on this point. Differential nerve blocks which impair conduction in myelinated fibres and are associated with the loss of only tactile sensibility frequently alleviate pain and hyperalgesia.[24,25] If large diameter afferent fibres are signalling pain, this implies some reorganisation in the central processing of somatosensory information. In some patients, however, hyperalgesia and pain only disappear during blockade of small diameter fibres.[26] A final important clinical finding is that pain will often radiate extensively beyond the area of damaged tissue or the innervation territory of the damaged nerve. The spread usually ignores traditional boundaries such as nerve territories or dermatomes. In extreme cases it can spread to encompass large areas of the body surface.[9] Occasionally, a 'mirror image' pain is apparent.[6] Again, these observations implicate changes within the central nervous system.

Many suggestions as to the cause of SMP involve the idea of a 'vicious circle' of events which are self-maintaining. A general scheme, which deliberately avoids reference to specific mechanisms, is shown in Figure 1. The initial precipitating cause, injury to peripheral tissues or nerves, may lead to some alteration in the functioning of primary sensory neurones, either as a direct response to injury or because of changes in the milieu in which the afferent nerve terminal lies. The afferent activity arising from the damaged periphery is signalled to the spinal cord where it is proposed that it distorts normal somatosensory processes, leading to excessive activity in ascending spinal systems concerned with the transmission of nociceptive information. The ability of peripheral inputs to produce just such a modification in the responses of dorsal horn neurones is documented by Wall (this issue). The altered central state is also held to be responsible for a modification in the responsiveness of sympathetic pre-ganglionics. The abnormal sympathetic activity produces the observed vasomotor, sudomotor and trophic changes in the peripheral tissues, and most importantly provides an element of positive feedback, reinforcing or exacerbating the abnormal sensory inflow. Direct recordings in man have not revealed that sympathetic efferents become hyperactive in these conditions.[27] However, animal experiments have shown that following peripheral nerve damage, the organisation of sympathetic reflexes is altered. Noticeably, the peripheral reflex control of sympathetic firing is qualitatively altered under these conditions.[28,29]

The presence of a feedback element in the scheme shown in Figure 1 has important implications. Control theory tells us that if the strength or gain of the feedback is sufficiently high, the system will be unstable and even small inputs will be amplified to produce an explosive afferent barrage. The system may also generate afferent input in the absence of sensory stimulation. If the gain of the feedback circuit is more modest it may be stable although still yielding large transient inputs to weak stimuli and a constant low level of ongoing input. Only if the feedback gain is sufficiently reduced will the system subside to become near-normal. Under this condition the system will be less sensitive to peripheral inputs and it will be more difficult to trigger large afferent barrages. It is

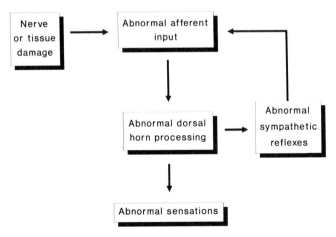

Fig. 1 A general scheme to explain how nerve injuries may lead to persistent sensory abnormalities.

also unlikely to produce ongoing inputs. It is interesting to note that causalgia patients often initially experience spontaneous pain and very developed hyperalgesia, and later have no spontaneous pain and a less sensitive hyperalgesia.[4] It is therefore tempting to suggest that in these patients the strength of the positive feedback, or its dynamics, are changing with time. In many patients, however, the pathophysiological state does not subside completely even over very prolonged periods. Wier Mitchell's son, also a neurologist, followed up 22 of his father's causalgia patients. After 20 years 16 were still in pain (see Ref. 30). Such a long time course of symptoms is consistent with the self-sustaining nature of the circuit shown in Figure 1.

Another important implication of the 'vicious circle' scheme proposed in Figure 1 is that some therapeutic benefit will derive from manoeuvres which reduce the feedback gain. One way of achieving this is to interfere with the ability of sympathetic efferents to activate sensory afferents. Various attempts in this direction have been made, but since the nature of the interaction, and even the type of afferent neurone responsible, are matters of dispute (see below) the most appropriate way to achieve this effect remains controversial. Similarly, a beneficial effect might be expected if one could block the alteration in central processing that leads to the abnormal patterns of sympathetic outflow. Unfortunately, the nature of these central disturbances is only now receiving detailed attention, and we presently have little information as to mechanisms (see Woolf, this issue).

One obvious practical way to break the vicious cycle of events depicted in Figure 1 is to open the feedback loop by cutting or blocking the sympathetic efferents. By definition this is effective in alleviating the pain in SMP. The sympathectomy can be achieved in a number of ways including surgical interruption or removal of the sympathetic chain, phenol or local anaesthetic blocks of sympathetic ganglia, or depletion of peripheral neurotransmitter stores by regional guanethidine treatment. In some cases the sympathectomy is reversible, which might be rapid or slow. Even transient blocks of sympathetic function may be of long term benefit by opening the feedback for sufficient time to allow the system to settle to some non-pathological level. If this occurs, even if sympathetic function in subsequently restored and the feedback loop is closed, there may be insufficient gain to drive the system to its previous explosive state.

One final observation one can make about the scheme shown in

Figure 1 is that it may be difficult to identify the initial or primary cause of the pathology. For instance, if the primary cause was the development of adrenosensitivity by nociceptive afferents, then normal sympathetic activity might activate those nociceptors which would reflexly drive sympathetic efferents at abnormal rates. Detailed examination of the system would reveal abnormalities in afferent and efferent function but it would be difficult to distinguish cause from effect. In fact, matters are likely to be even more confusing. In the example given above, the increased nociceptor activity we postulated to occur might not only slavishly drive sympathetic neurones to fire excessively, but also produce qualitative changes in the response properties of other neuronal elements. It would then become exceedingly difficult to pinpoint the primary cause in the interacting abnormalities. For this reason it is perhaps not surprising that there are multiple suggestions as to the primary disturbance in SMP. Each of these has its pundits, and each has some clinical or laboratory findings in its favour. However, none on its own offers an explanation of all the observed properties of SMP's.

SPECIFIC HYPOTHESES AS TO THE PRIMARY CAUSE OF SMP

Whilst the search for mechanisms has arisen from the existence of SMP states in patients, detailed studies have relied heavily upon animal studies and animal models. The most studied preparation is the rat neuroma model in which a major peripheral nerve (usually the sciatic) is simply tightly ligated and cut distally. The cut axons form multiple sprouts which would normally initiate efforts at regeneration, but they are unable to escape from the end of the cut nerve and so develop into a swollen neuroma. Whilst this preparation is easily and reproducibly made, it is not clear just how well it models the clinical disorders. On the one hand, rats so treated behave as if they have some neurogenic pain,[31] whilst on the other, only a small proportion of patients with similar complete nerve lesions develop painful sequelae. In the past few years there have been efforts to develop new animal models that involve only partial nerve damage, created by ligating only part of a major nerve or loosely constricting the nerve so that its subsequent swelling produces a partial demyelination and degeneration in the nerve.[32,33] Behaviourial observations indicate that these may indeed reflect more accurately the symptoms of patients. These animals are also improved by sympathectomy. But to date the type of pathophysiology that has been seen in these new models is similar to that reported for the neuroma model.

The experimental work has focused on changes that occur in the periphery and changes that occur in the dorsal horn.

Peripheral changes

Ephaptic connections

One possibility is that structural changes in the nerve allow axons to become very closely associated[34] and for cross-talk to develop between them. The suggestion is that electrical activity in one axon terminal may excite an adjacent axon not via the release of neurotransmitter but by the direct flow of current. If multiple ephapses occur, they could have the effect of magnifying aberrant impulses. However, the experimental evidence does not suggest that this mechanism is an important one. In rat and monkey neuromata few ephapses are seen and they are only found at long post-injury times (whilst symptoms in patients can appear rapidly).[28,35] Moreover, to date they have only been observed between sensory fibres and not between sympathetic and sensory axons. Thus, whilst this mechanism could explain a component of the hyperalgesia experienced by many patients, it offers no explanation for the sympathetic dependency of the pain state or of the radiation of symptoms beyond the territory of an injured nerve.

Adrenergic receptors on primary sensory neurones

The observations of Wall & Gutnick,[36,37] that many unmyelinated and myelinated afferent fibres innervating a rat neuroma were excited by adrenalin and noradrenaline, raised the possibility that the damaged fibres came to express adrenoreceptors. Much subsequent work, reviewed by Devor in this issue, has confirmed that appreciable numbers of damaged fibres in a variety of species show this sensitivity. Moreover, there is now good evidence that normal levels of sympathetic firing can activate some damaged afferents.[38] Interestingly, Devor & Raber have also shown[39,40] that some strains of rat are much more prone to develop this abnormality, raising the possibility that only some individuals (with the appropriate genetic make-up) will be likely to acquire SMP. Whilst this suggestion offers an explanation for the low incidence of SMP in patients with apparently similar lesions, it is confounded by the clinical observation that in those patients unfortunate enough to suffer two similar nerve injuries, pain and hyperalgesia are not usually a present in both.[30] In all experimental studies of damaged nerves the effects of adrenergic agents appeared to be mediated by α-receptors. Similarly in patients, regional blockade with the alpha-adrenergic antagonist phentolamine is as effective as local anaesthetic block of sympathetic ganglia in relieving pain and hyperalgesia.[41] The simplest explanation of these effects is that damaged sensory neurones, particularly nociceptive neurones, up-regulate their expression of α-receptors. We have studied this possibility directly by examining the binding of clonidine to intact and damaged rat sciatic nerve (Small, Priestley, Scadding and McMahon, in preparation). Figure 2 shows autoradiographs of the distribution of binding sites in the nerve and dorsal horn obtained from rats with 3 week-old neuromata. Counting of grain densities from a number of similar preparations revealed a consistent and significant elevation of binding sites in the neuroma and in the superficial dorsal horn where many unmyelinated afferents are known to terminate. These data support the suggestion that damaged sensory neurones can increase their expression of adrenoreceptors. Unfortunately the limited resolution of the technique has not allowed us determine if small and/or large DRG cells show this change.

The presence of adrenoreceptors on nociceptive terminals would provide a ready explanation for the ability of sympathetic activity to produce pain in man. It is less clear how it might itself explain the hyperalgesia that is so common in SMP (and which is usually concomitantly relieved by sympathetic block). It also offers no explanation for the radiation of symptoms to normal tissue.

Indirect coupling of sympathetic and sensory fibres

In addition to the direct chemical coupling between sympathetic and sensory neurones, there is the possibility of indirect effects in which efferent sympathetic activity precipitates a cascade of chemical changes in the microenvironment surrounding the axon terminals, perhaps leading to the production of other agents which excite or sensitize afferent endings. One reason for making this suggestion is that the effects of adrenergic agents on damaged sensory nerve terminals often have a surprisingly long latency, sometimes in the order of tens of seconds.[39] Another reason is that

there is recent pharmacological evidence from several other experimental models of painful or hyperalgesic states demonstrating just
such a complex series of changes induced by sympathetic activity

A.

B.

C.

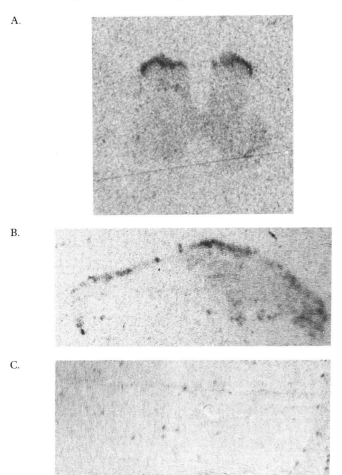

Fig. 2 Photomicrographs of spinal cord (**A**) and peripheral nerve (**B** & **C**) showing
the binding of radiolabelled clonidine. (**A**) shows a 30 micron transverse section
of spinal cord taken from the 5th lumbar segment. The sciatic nerve had been cut
on the left hand side 3 weeks previously. There is an increase in the binding of
clonidine on this side, particularly in the superficial dorsal horn. Densimetric
measurements showed a significant (70%) increase in binding in the superficial
dorsal horn on the side of nerve section. (**B**) shows the binding of clonidine in a
longitudinal section of a rat sciatic nerve which had been cut 3 weeks previously.
The neuroma, on the right of the section, shows high levels of clonidine binding.
In comparison, similarly treated sections of acutely cut nerves showed no significant labelling. An example is shown in (**C**).

in damaged but not normal skin.[22,42-44] The findings from these studies are summarised in Figure 3. One proposed mechanism is that adrenergic agents released from postganglionic neurones activate autoreceptors on the same terminals, stimulating them to release prostaglandins. Bradykinin may also act in a similar indirect fashion, although producing different prostaglandins. The prostaglandins are then proposed to sensitize the terminals of otherwise normal nociceptive afferents, leading to hyperalgesia. A second indirect mechanism involves another byproduct of arachidonic acid metabolism, leukotriene B4, which appears able to attract and then stimulate polymorphonuclear leukocytes to produce an algogen which also directly activates nociceptive terminals, dihydroxyeicosa-tetraenoic acid-(diHETE). Since the formation of diHETE is insensitive to the blocking actions of NSAIDs, such as indomethacin (and as SMP also appears resistant to these agents), perhaps it is an important contributor to SMP. However, there is to date no direct evidence for such a suggestion. Whilst the models may explain the pain and hyperalgesia of SMP, and the beneficial effects of sympathectomy, they do not explain the radiation of pain. There are two other problems. Firstly, the

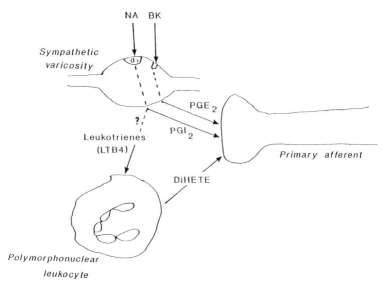

Fig. 3 Indirect mechanisms leading to the excitation or sensitization of nociceptive terminals in damaged tissue, based on observations on animal models of hyperalgesia (*see text* for details).

effects of adrenergic agents are believed to be mediated by α_2 receptors in these models, whereas α_1 antagonists are reportedly effective at relieving the hyperalgesia and pain in SMP.[41] Secondly, Wallin et al.[7] reported experiments on a small number of patients in which they found that iontophoresis of noradrenaline could rekindle pain in causalgia patients (but not normal subjects), including some who had previously been subjected to a sympathectomy, i.e. without postganglionic axons to participate as described above. In view of the key importance of these findings it would be interesting if these preliminary experiments were repeated.

Sensitization of nociceptive afferents

One final proposal is that the primary cause of symptoms in reflex sympathetic dystrophy is the injury-induced sensitization of nociceptive afferents, and in this scheme sympathetic efferents play only a secondary role. In one carefully studied patient Cline et al.[26] observed pain and hyperalgesia which was not relieved by A-fibre peripheral nerve blocks (cf.[24,25]) but which did disappear with total nerve block. Microneurographic recordings revealed C fibres with lower than normal mechanical thresholds and yielding long after discharges to brief stimuli. These workers suggested that in this and perhaps other patients, the aberrant responsiveness of nociceptors might have been triggered by the initial tissue or nerve injury, but then have become self-sustaining if antidromic impulses in terminal branches of the nociceptors were capable of further sensitizing the afferents. Sensitization of peripheral terminals of nociceptors to thermal but not mechanical stimuli has been reported following antidromic activity in some[45] but not all[46,47] animal experiments. Antidromic activity in C sensory neurones can induce vasodilation, and if this can be maintained chronically (which may not be the case) this might contribute to the vasomotor disturbances seen in patients. Thus a vicious circle of sensitization-activity-sensitization might exist entirely within the nociceptive neurone, although the evidence for such a mechanism remains entirely circumstantial. Sympathetic efferents could exacerbate the condition either by altering skin temperature and thus activating thermally sensitized nociceptors (although at least some patients' pains are improved by cooling) or by activating sensitized nociceptors (a suggestion for which there is some experimental support[14,20,21]).

This proposal, like all other explanations which place the primary abnormality in the periphery, suffers from an inability to explain the frequently observed radiation of pain, and the ability of activity in large A fibres to produce pain in many patients.

Central changes

The ability of peripheral nerve lesions or peripheral tissue injury to alter spinal somatosensory processes is becoming well recognized and is reviewed by Wall in this issue. The ascending spinal pathways that transmit information rostrad begin to respond more vigorously to peripheral inputs, and indeed can become responsive to totally new inputs that normally do not drive them. These cells also relay aberrant activity generated from the periphery. This process can develop quite rapidly with peripheral tissue injury, and it is possible that once established it may become largely independent of the precipitating event.[48] A second type of disturbance is seen in the response properties and patterns of reflex organization in the sympathetic nervous system, as described above. Within the dorsal horn, the representation of the body surface is very compressed, especially in the mediolateral plane. Expansion of receptive fields over quite substantial areas of the body surface are therefore possible and provide an explanation for the radiation of pain.

One specific hypothesis was advanced recently by Roberts (1986) which is illustrated in Figure 4. In this model, the activity generated in nociceptors by the initial injury is held to produce a sensitization of dorsal horn output cells. After this initial event, all the pathology is placed in the CNS. Activity in large afferent A-fibres will excessively excite the sensitized dorsal horn cells. Sympathetic efferents can produce a small excitation of normal, undamaged tactile afferents (see above) and this, it is suggested, contributes to the pain state. Whilst this hypothesis rather neatly explains many of the sensory disturbances solely on the basis of sensitized dorsal horn cells, it is deficient in at least one respect— it does not adequately explain the ability of sympathectomy to relieve abnormal skin sensitivity! For whilst sympathectomy would prevent these efferents activating mechanosensitive afferents, it would not prevent light mechanical stimuli from exciting them. And one common finding in patients is that hyperalgesia is immediately relieved by sympathectomy. Additionally, such an hypothesis cannot be readily applied to cases of complete nerve

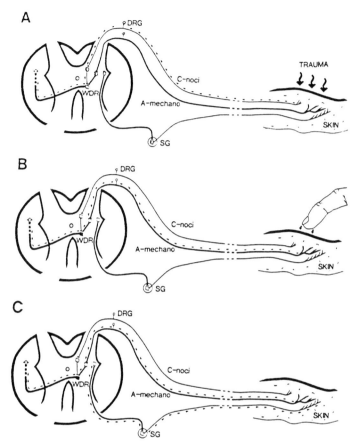

Fig. 4 Schematic diagram of a hypothesis of the pathophysiology in SMP. (**A**) illustrates the immediate response to cutaneous trauma. Action potentials in C-nociceptors propogate through the dorsal root ganglion (DRG) to the spinal cord where they activate and sensitize wide-dynamic-range (WDR) neurones whose axons ascend to higher centres. In **B**, the WDR neurones remain sensitized and now respond to activity in large diameter A-mechanoreceptors which are activated by light touch. In **C**, the same sensitized WDR neurones respond again to A-mechanoreceptors, but this is initiated by sympathetic efferent actions on the sensory receptor, in the absence of cutaneous stimulation. This phase represents sympathetically maintained pain. (*From:* Roberts WJ. A hypothesis on the physiological basis for causalgia and related pain, PAIN 24; 1986: 297–311. Reproduced with permission.).

transection where there is no mechanism for generating A-fibre discharges (other than by peripheral pathophysiology—which is excluded in this model).

From the foregoing description it would appear that hypotheses based entirely on either peripheral or central abnormalities are unable to explain adequately all the disturbances seen in all patients with peripheral nerve injuries. This is perhaps not surprising since it is clear that an abnormality at one locus frequently leads to changes at another. The existence of multiple pathophysiologies co-existing in a single patient is therefore not to be unexpected. On the other hand, it is likely that different pathologies will be dominant in different patients. And indeed the heterogeneity of pathologies expressed by patients may limit the effectiveness of therapies aimed at only one locus. It is feasible that detailed laboratory testing could be used to determine the relative contribution of different pathophysiological mechanisms in individual patients.

REFERENCES

1 Mitchell SW, Morehouse GR, Keen WW. Injuries of nerves and their consequences. Philadelphia: JB Lippincott, 1864
2 Wall PD. The hyperpathic syndrome: A challenge to specificity theory. In: von Euler C, Franzen O, Londblom U, Ottoson D, eds. Somatosensory mechanisms. Wenner-Gren International symposium. London: MacMillan, 1984; Vol. 41: pp. 327–337
3 Schott GD. Mechanisms of causalgia and related clinical conditions. The role of the sympathetic nervous system. Brain 1986; 109: 717–738
4 Janig W, Kollmann W. The involvement of the sympathetic nervous system in pain. Drug Res 1984; 34: 1066-1–73
5 Livingston WK. Pain mechanisms, a physiological interpretation of causalgia and its related states. New York: MacMillan, 1943; pp. 83–127
6 Loh L, Nathan PW. Painful peripheral states and sympathetic blocks. J Neurol Neurosurg Psychiat 1978; 41: 664–671
7 Wallin G, Torebjork E, Hallin R. Preliminary observations on the pathophysiology of hyperalgesia in the causalgic pain syndrome. In: Zotterman Y, ed. Sensory functions of the skin in primates with special reference to man. Oxford: Pergamon. 1976; pp. 489–502
8 Roberts WJ, Elardo SM. Sympathetic activation of unmyelinated mechanoreceptors in cat skin. Brain Res 1985; 339: pp. 123–125
9 Nathan PW. Pain and the sympathetic nervous system. J Auton Nerv Syst 1983; 7: pp. 363–370
10 Frost SA, Raja SN, Campbell JN, Meyer RA, Khan AA. Does hyperalgesia to cooling stimuli characterize patients with sympathetically maintained pain (reflex sympathetic dystrophy)? In: Dubner R, Gebhart GF, Bond MR, eds. Proceedings of the Vth world congress on pain. Amsterdam: Elsevier, 1988; pp. 151–156
11 Wynn Parry CB, Withrington RH. Painful disorders of peripheral nerves. Postgrad Med J 1984; 60: pp. 869–875
12 Akoev GN. Catecholamines, acetylycholine and excitability of mechanoreceptors. Prog Neurobiol 1980; 15: pp. 269–294
13 Davies SN. Sympathetic stimulation causes a frequency dependent excitation and suppression of thermoreceptive cells in the trigeminal nucleus of the rat. J Physiol 1984; 350: pp. 22P

14 Roberts WJ, Elardo SM. Sympathetic activation of unmyelinated mechanoreceptors in cat skin. Brain Res 1985; 339: pp. 123–125
15 Barasi S, Lynn B. Effects of sympathetic stimulation on mechanoreceptive and nociceptive afferent units from the rabbit pinna. Brain Res 1986; 378: pp. 21–27
16 Pierce TP, Roberts WJ. Sympathetically induced changes in the responses of gaurd hairs and type II receptors in the cat. J Physiol 1981; 314: pp. 411–428
17 Roberts WJ, Foglesong ME. Identification of afferents contributing to sympathetically evoked activity in wide-dynamic range neurons. Pain 1988; 34: pp. 305–314
18 Roberts WJ, Elardo SM, King KA. Sympathetically-induced changes in the responses of slowly-adapting type I receptors in cat skin. Somatosens Res 1985; 2: pp. 223–236
19 Shea VK, Perl ER. Failure of sympathetic stimulation to affect responsiveness of rabbit polymodal nociceptors. J Neurophysiol 1985; 54: pp. 513–519
20 Sanjue H, Jun Z. Sympathetic facilitation of sustained discharges of polymodal nociceptors. Pain 1989; 38: pp. 85–90
21 Sato J, Perl ER. Sympathetic activation increases nociceptor responses after nerve injury. Soc Neurosci Abs 1989; 15: 176.12
22 Levine JD, Tairo YO, Collins SD, Tam JK. Noradrenaline hyperalgesia is mediated through interaction with sympathetic postganlionic neurone terminals rather than activation of primary afferent nociceptors. Nature 1986; 323: pp. 158–169
23 Lewis T. Pain. New York: Macmillan, 1942
24 Campbell JN, Raja SN, Meyer RA. Painful sequelae of nerve injury. In: R Dubner, GF Gebhart, MR Bond, eds. Proceedings of the Vth world congress on Pain. Amsterdam: Elsevier, 1988; pp. 135–143
25 Campbell JN, Raja SN, Meyer RA, MacKinnon SE. Myelinated afferents signal the hyperalgesia associated with nerve injury. Pain 1988; 32: pp. 89–94
26 Cline MA, Ochoa J, Torebjork E. Chronic hyperalgesia and skin warming caused by sensitized C nociceptors. Brain 1989; 112: pp. 621–647
27 Janig W. The sympathetic nervous system in pain: Physiology and Pathophysiology. In: Stanton-Hicks M, ed. Pain and the sympathetic nervous system. London: Kluwer, 1989; pp. 17–89
28 Blumberg H, Janig W. Reflex patterns in postganglionic vasoconstrictor neurones following chronic nerve lesions. J Auton Nerv Syst 1985; 14: pp. 157–180
29 Koltzenburg M. Sympathetic reflexes change when cutaneous nerves of the adult cat re-innervate inappropriate target tissue. J Physiol 1989; 414: 34P
30 Nathan PW. The sympathetic system and pain. Funct Neurol 1989; 4: 11–15
31 Wall PD, Devor M, Inbal R, Scadding JW, Schonfeld D. Autonomy following peripheral nerve lesions: experimental anaesthesia dolorosa. Pain 1979; 7: pp. 103–113
32 Bennett GJ, Xie YK. An experimental peripheral neuropathy in rat that produces abnormal pain sensations. In: R Dubner, GF Gebhart, MR Bond, eds. Proceedings of the Vth world congress on Pain. Amsterdam: Elsevier 1988; pp. 129–134
33 Selzer Z, Shir Y. Lack of sensitization of primary afferent receptors by prostaglandins in a rat model of causalgic chronic pains. Agents Actions 1988; 25: pp. 252–254
34 Bernstein JJ, Pagnanelli D. Long-term axonal apposition in rat sciatic nerve neuroma. J Neurosurg 1982; 57: pp. 682–684
35 Meyer RA, Raja SN, Campbell JN, MacKinnon SE. Neuronal activity originating from a neuroma in the baboon. Brain Res 1985; 325: pp. 255–260
36 Wall PD, Gutnick M. Ongoing activity in peripheral nerves: The physiology and pharmacology of impulses originating from a neuroma. Exp Neurol 1974; 43: pp. 580–593

37 Wall PD, Gutnick M. Properties of afferent nerve impulses originating from a neuroma. Nature 1974; 248: pp. 740–743

38 Habler HJ, Janig W, Koltzenburg M. Activation of unmyelinated afferents in chronically lesioned nerves by adrenaline and excitation of sympathetic efferents in the cat. Neuro Sci Lett 1987; 82: pp. 35–40

39 Devor M. The pathophysiology and anatomy of damaged nerve. In: PD Wall, R Melzack, eds. Textbook of Pain (2nd Ed). Edinburgh: Churchill Livingstone, pp. 63–81

40 Devor M, Raber P. Heritability of symptoms in an experimental model of neuropathic pain. Pain 1990; 42: pp. 51–67

41 Trede R-D, Raja SN, Davis KD, Meyer RA, Campbell JN. Evidence that alpha-adrenergic receptors mediate sympathetically maintained pain (reflex sympathetic dystrophy). Pain 1990; Suppl. 5: p. 944

42 Taiwo YO, Levine JD. Characterization of the arachidonic acid metabolites mediating bradykinin and noradrenalin hyperalgesia. Brain Res 1988; 458: pp. 402–406

43 Levine JD, Lau W, Kwait G, Goetzl EJ. Leukotriene B4 produces hyperalgesia that is dependent on polymorphonuclear leukocytes. Science 1984; 225: pp. 743–745

44 Coderre TJ, Basbaum AI, Levine JD. Neural control of vascular permeability: interactions between primary afferents, mast cells, and sympathetic efferents. J Neurophysiol 1989; 62: pp. 48–58

45 Fitzgerald M. The spread of sensitization of polymodal nociceptors in the rabbit from nearby injury and by antidromic nerve stimulation. J Physiol 1979; 297: pp. 207–216

46 Reeh PW, Kocher L, Jung S. Does neurogenic inflammation alter the sensitivity of unmyelinated nociceptors in the rat? Brain Res 1986; 384: pp. 42–50

47 Meyer RA, Campbell JN, Raja SN. Antidromic nerve stimulation in the monkey does not sensitize unmyelinated nociceptors to heat. Brain Res 1988; 441: pp. 168–172

48 McMahon SB, Wall PD. Receptive fields of rat lamina I projection cells move to incorporate a region of nearby injury. Pain 1984; 19: pp. 235–247

British Medical Bulletin (1991) Vol. 47, No. 3, pp. 601–618

Management of sympathetic pain

J E Charlton
Pain Management Service, Royal Victoria Infirmary, Newcastle upon Tyne, UK

Successful treatment of sympathetic pain is directed at the restoration of normal function. This can be achieved in the majority of cases with a combination of appropriate sympathetic or somatic nerve block, usually coupled with aggressive physiotherapy. It is a matter of regret that there are few controlled trials to demonstrate the efficacy of any of these forms of management.

Other non-invasive techniques such as stimulation-produced analgesia and pharmacology, particularly the use of adrenergic blocking agents, hold some promise of future benefit. Here too, more effort should be made to carry out properly designed studies, as there is scepticism about the place of permanent or potentially destructive therapy in any painful condition.

This chapter considers sympathetic pain and should be read in conjunction with the chapter on mechanisms of sympathetic pain by McMahon. Changes in the terminology concerning conditions that present with the signs and symptoms of sympathetic overactivity are occurring in response to increasing knowledge of the underlying mechanisms. Such pain is now known as sympathetically-maintained pain. The most widely known examples of sympathetically maintained pain are **causalgia** and **reflex sympathetic dystrophy**. For the purposes of this chapter all clinical conditions presenting with an element of sympathetic overactivity will be regarded as being part of the same process.

The *International Association for the Study of Pain* has suggested that reflex sympathetic dystrophy be defined as, 'Continuous pain in a portion of an extremity which may include fracture but does not involve a major nerve, and is associated with sympathetic hyperactivity'. Causalgia, which by definition involves neural injury is defined separately, but the sense of this approach is arguable since the symptoms, clinical presentation and treatment all overlap, thus suggesting a common pathophysiology.

DEFINITIONS

More recently a definition of reflex sympathetic dystrophy has been proposed which encompasses the varying clinical presentations:

> 'A syndrome of continuous diffuse limb pain, often burning in nature, and usually consequent to injury or noxious stimulus, and disuse, presenting with variable sensory, motor, autonomic and trophic changes; causalgia represents a specific presentation of reflex sympathetic dystrophy associated with a peripheral nerve injury.'[1]

CLINICAL FEATURES

The symptoms and changes spread independently of both the source and site of the precipitating event. Clinical findings include disturbances of:

Autonomic regulation. Alterations in blood flow, hyper- or hypohidrosis, oedema. There may be changes to skin, hair and nails.

Sensation. Hyper or hypoaesthesia, allodynia to cold and mechanical stimulation.

Motor function. Weakness, tremor, joint stiffness.

Psychologic function. These are the same reactive changes that may occur with any pain patient and may include anxiety, depression and hopelessness.

These features may present diffusely, but not necessarily uniformly, in the entire distal extremity. They occur at a variable time after the onset of the syndrome, spreading proximally in a glove and stocking distribution that is not associated with a dermatome or peripheral nerve. Classically, dominant symptoms are spontaneous burning pain, swelling and weakness, and it is reasonable to regard all burning pain as being sympathetically maintained until proved otherwise. However, cases may present with marked differences in pain intensity and clinical features. These differences are frequently unrelated to the precipitating cause or to the time since the injury. The diagnosis may be missed by those unfamiliar with the syndrome because of the non-anatomic, diffuse nature of the clinical presentation. As the disease process progresses, the pain may take on an aching quality especially when it involves limb girdles and other limbs.

AIDS TO DIAGNOSIS

Patients presenting with sympathetically maintained pain should be graded according to severity of their presentation in each category. Thus, they should be graded as mild, moderate or severe in each of the categories of sensory, autonomic or motor change. Careful assessment in each category will help diagnosis.

Autonomic function. Bilateral symmetrical multidigital temperature measurement by surface thermistors or by thermography, show consistent differences on the affected side, which may be cooler or warmer, or both in turn.

Sensory function. Lowered thresholds to pinprick, light touch and cold.

Motor function. Reduced strength and range of movement to active and passive testing.

Response to neural blockade. Sympathetic block usually abolishes the diffuse burning pain and the allodynia. It abolishes the vasoconstrictor response to cold stimulation.

Bone scan. Three phase bone scanning shows distinctive, diffuse patterns of increased flow, pooling and delay.

There are other non-specific tests which can be used to measure change and response to treatment. These may include measurement of bone density by radiography, water displacement plethysmography for measures of swelling, and tests of sudomotor function, such as skin conductivity and quantitative sweat testing.

CATEGORIES OF SYMPATHETIC PAIN

Stage 1 (mild)

Beginning within days to a few weeks of the precipitating event, this stage is characterized by pain, often burning, at the site of the injury. This may be accompanied by allodynia. The limb is held immobile and there is accompanying oedema, tenderness and local muscle spasm. The limb may be warm, red and dry, or cool and pale. At this stage the disease may resolve spontaneously or respond rapidly to appropriate treatment. The duration of this clinical picture may last from days to months.

Stage 2 (moderate)

As the disease process progresses, the pain can be increased, decreased or unchanged. Sensation may be markedly altered and associated with local swelling, joint stiffness and muscle wasting in the area of the injury. Changes distant to the site of injury are seen and the affected limb is cold, moist and may vary in colour from pale to cyanotic. Osteoporosis is becoming diffuse and increased technetium uptake by scintigraphy is seen. Treatment can still be effective but the response is attenuated and symptoms may persist for many months.

Stage 3 (severe)

Severe trophic changes are present and these changes are very resistant to any form of treatment. The pain is constant and now has an additional aching and throbbing component. The affected limb is cold, damp and virtually immobile secondary to joint and muscle contractures. Skin and subcutaneous tissues are atrophied and appear smooth, thin and shiny. Hair and nails are coarse, thickened and brittle. Radiologically, a diffuse osteoporosis is present. Psychologic and psychiatric abnormalities may be present. The changes seen may be permanent and treatment is unlikely to help.

INCIDENCE AND EPIDEMIOLOGY

Little is known concerning the overall incidence of sympathetically maintained pain in the general population. Abram has estimated that the overall incidence of causalgia and reflex sympathetic dystrophy seen in a pain clinic population varies between 6 and 11%.[2] The list of conditions that have been known to trigger the process of sympathetically maintained pain is extensive and includes sprains, fractures, lacerations, crush injuries, amputations and burns. It may follow surgery and occupational factors, such as repetitive microtrauma and pneumatic tool operation, and it has been reported after many medical conditions such as myocardial infarction, neurologic diseases, infection and vascular disease.

Blunt trauma, strain/sprain, crush and blast injuries are the usual cause. The syndrome may be seen with or without an associated fracture. The ratio of males to females varies with reported series. Abram and others reported that about 60% of patients with sympathetic pain were female.[2-4] In other series males have outnumbered females by 2:1,[5] or represented 55% of those seen.[6] The latter paper also noted a low incidence among black patients. Rothberg et al. described a higher incidence of sympathetically maintained pain in patients over the age of 35,[7] and this was noted in the reports of Pak[3] and Kleinert,[6] who suggest that most cases occur between the ages of 35 to 60, with few cases occurring in patients under 30 or over 70.

This is not to say that the condition is never seen in children. It may be that it is more common than has been supposed until now. Abram has reviewed the literature and has found over 100 case reports.[2] There are insufficient data for a clear clinical picture to be presented, but it appears to be more common in females and to involve the lower limb most frequently. Few cases involve antecedent trauma, although antecedent stress and anxiety was present on numerous occasions. Cases as young as three years of age have occurred and most have responded well to normal therapy.

The term causalgia has been associated classically with injury to a nerve trunk. In these circumstances the majority follow gunshot wounds, most of which are proximal to the knee or elbow. The majority of cases are related to partial transsections of the medial cord of the brachial plexus, the median nerve or the sciatic nerve. However, problems have been reported following injury to virtually any sensory nerve in the body. The review carried out by Schwartzman and McLellan cites an incidence of between 1 and 15% among nerve injured patients.[8] The overall incidence appears to be around 4%[9] with about 20% reporting at least transient symptoms of sympathetically maintained pain.[10]

PRINCIPLES OF TREATMENT

The underlying principle of the management of any chronic painful process is the restoration of normal function. All efforts in the management of sympathetically maintained pain should be directed towards this goal. There is no single therapy that can be guaranteed to be effective and the rehabilitation of virtually all patients will require multiple therapeutic interventions. Equally, evaluation of treatment is made more difficult by the complex and varying presentation of the condition. In general the first line of treatment will consist of treatment of the precipitating injury, followed by sympathetic blockade and aggressive active and passive physiotherapy.

Treatment of the precipitating injury

It is axiomatic that treatment of the local injury takes precedence over active physiotherapy. This includes treatment at the site of the injury and the relief of acute pain. Proper care of the local injury may require debridement, removal of foreign bodies, adequate reduction and decompression of fractures, surgical correction of torn muscles, tendons and ligaments, early repair of neural injury and active treatment of any infection. The use of regional anaesthetic techniques may be particularly appropriate in this context as it may lead to less postoperative pain.[11] It is interesting to speculate whether the increased use of regional techniques for trauma surgery would lead to a reduced incidence of sympathetic pain and other chronic painful sequelae as has been described for phantom limb and stump pain after amputation.[12,13]

SYMPATHETIC NERVE BLOCKS

Diagnostic blocks

It is mandatory that diagnostic blockade be carried out on any patient suspected of having a sympathetically maintained pain. Delay in diagnosis can lead to delay in appropriate treatment. When performing diagnostic blockade it is important to recall the basic principles concerned. Every patient should have a full interview and examination recorded. If sympathetic pain is suspected, the evaluation of the presenting features described earlier is most important to provide baselines for assessment of the response to diagnostic blockade and to treatment.

The purposes of diagnostic nerve block in the management of chronic pain are as follows:[14]

1. To diagnose the site of the pain.
2. To identify the contribution from the sympathetic nervous system.

3. To separate somatic from visceral pain.
4. To separate local disease from referred pain.
5. To distinguish peripheral nerve from dermatomal input.
6. To aid in the diagnosis of 'centrally-generated' pain disorders.
7. To prognosticate further therapeutic procedures.

Prior to diagnostic blockade the patient should have their 'normal' pain pattern and the effect of the block should be rigorously assessed in the light of the previous examination. For the most reliable results it is recommended that a small volume of a long-acting agent be used, and that the block be performed using a nerve stimulator to permit precise localization of the target nerve. If a block has been successful the following principles apply:[14]

1. There may be a subjective response, i.e. the patient feels better.
2. There may be an improvement in the function of the blocked area.
3. These improvements should be associated with objective evidence that the block is working, with appropriate sensory, motor or sympathetic changes. (For tests of sympathetic function see Lofstrom and Cousins[15])
4. The time course of the block usually should be appropriate to the agent employed.

A positive response to a block may be due to other reasons than a successful nerve block. The commonest reason is placebo response, which may occur in up to 40% of patients.[16] This is **not** evidence of a psychological aetiology. Placebo response is a normal response that tends to diminish with repeated exposure to a stimulus, and thus reduced rather than increased benefit will be seen with repeated blocks. There may be other reasons for false positive and false negative responses to nerve blocks and these have been summarized by Charlton.[14] It should be recognized also that the therapeutic result may outlast the clinical effect of the block by a considerable margin. This too, must be regarded as a normal response for which we have, as yet, no explanation.[17,18]

Therapeutic blocks

It should be re-emphasized again that sympathetic blockade alone will not relieve the problems caused by sympathetically maintained pain. Perhaps the most important point that can be made is that the patient must accept a great responsibility for their own care.

As disuse and loss of normal function appear to play an important part in the genesis of the clinical problem, it follows that resumption of activity is essential to sustain relief and promote ultimate resolution. Sympathetic blockade merely interrupts the painful cycle and permits the resumption of normal activity.

Sympathetic blockade may produce a pain-free period, and this should be used to undertake regular, active physiotherapy. Boas has suggested that activity should be pursued to the point of obsession, 'several minutes on the hour, every hour'.[19] He makes the most important point that reliance on sympathetic block alone will be insufficient to achieve a lasting cure, especially where there are advanced tissue changes secondary to long-standing disease. In these latter cases somatic nerve block may allow more complete relief of pain and allow for more aggressive therapy.

TECHNIQUES OF SYMPATHETIC BLOCK

Stellate ganglion block

Classical approaches to the stellate ganglion are to be found in any standard textbook.[15,20] Most of these advocate an approach to the cervical sympathetic chain at the level of C6, arguing that a lower approach carries with it an unacceptable risk of pneumothorax. An advance on these standard methods is contained in the modification described by Racz,[21] whereby the needle is angled more medially than in the classical description. This means that the needle will make contact with the body of the vertebra rather than the transverse process. This will reduce the hazards of hitting pleura if the needle is being inserted at the level of C7, and reduce the likelihood of accidental puncture of the vertebral artery if the needle is being inserted at either C6 or C7.

The point of entry of the needle is important as insertion of the needle at C7 permits the use of smaller volumes of solution and gives a more caudal spread, thus giving a greater certainty of blocking the sympathetics to the arm. Close monitoring, the use of a test dose and an isolated needle as described by Winnie,[22] are all aids to safety which must be adhered to no matter which technique is employed. It is possible to block other structures such as recurrent laryngeal nerve, phrenic nerve and brachial plexus, and rarely there may be subarachnoid or epidural spread, thus this is not a block to be undertaken lightly. Adequate spread of solution to effect a good block of the arm can be achieved with volumes of between 10 and 15 ml of local anaesthetic.

Neurolytic blockade of the stellate ganglion has been reported to be successful in the management of sympathetic pain.[15,21] However, this procedure is not without risk and, as described later, is not 'permanent'. Alternative techniques such as intravenous regional sympathetic block, stimulation techniques or drugs should be considered if long term relief is not being achieved with serial neural blockade.

Lumbar sympathetic block

Single needle approaches, with the patient lying on their side or in the prone position, and with needle placement at either L2 or L3 will yield a very high success rate. The technique described by the Auckland group,[23] has been shown to be effective and provide good spread of solution over two or three segments; more than enough for a successful block. The approach should be made some 8–10 cm from the midline as this will permit the best angle of attack to make contact with the sympathetic chain. A more sagittal angle of insertion will increase the risk of injury to genitofemoral nerve by permitting spread of solution laterally into the psoas sheath. There is an increased likelihood of penetrating the kidney with a more lateral approach, but this has not been shown to carry any risk. Correctly placed, volumes of 10 to 15 ml of local anaesthetic solution will give an adequate block using a single needle technique.

Drug choice

Local anaesthetic

Choice of local anaesthetic agent is only important during the initial diagnostic blockade for the reasons stated previously. Once the block is established the therapeutic effects may outlast drug action itself by a large amount. Thus it is possible to reduce potential problems by using safer local anaesthetic drugs such as lignocaine or prilocaine.

Neurolytic agents

Radiologic control is mandatory for every neurolytic block except under the most exceptional circumstances. There are almost no reports of the use of alcohol for either stellate ganglion or lumbar sympathetic block. Reports of neurolytic block of the stellate ganglion are rare. Where the use of phenol has been described, 1 to 2 ml of 10% phenol in contrast, with the addition of 40 mg of Depo-medrone and 1 to 2 ml of local anaesthetic, is the preferred solution. This volume will probably be insufficient to guarantee spread to the sympathetic outflow to the arm, and the use of larger volumes of this mixture may well be associated with spread onto other structures.

Phenol in contrast is the drug of choice for neurolytic block of the lumbar sympathetic chain. This is appropriate where serial blockade with local anaesthetic or alternative methods have failed to obtain prolonged pain relief and resolution of symptoms. Phenol solutions in contrast media are stable and safe.[24] Phenol block is not 'permanent', and provides extended blockade at best, as nerve regeneration has been shown to occur over a matter of weeks.[25]

Intravenous regional sympathetic blocks

The introduction of the intravenous sympathetic regional block using guanethidine in 1974 was accepted uncritically as a long lasting alternative to formal sympathetic blockade.[26] The technique has been described extensively by the author,[27] and consists of isolating the affected limb with a tourniquet inflated to a pressure in excess of the systolic blood pressure, and then injecting an intravenous dose of guanethidine to perfuse the limb by back diffusion. The guanethidine is strongly bound to sympathetic nerve endings and, as a false transmitter of noradrenaline, will displace noradrenaline from the pre-synaptic vesicles and prevent its re-uptake.

The normal dose of guanethidine is 15 to 20 mg of guanethidine in a carrier of 25–40 ml of normal saline depending upon the size of the limb to be blocked. The injection is painful and a small dose of local anaesthetic may help to reduce the pain. The tourniquet should remain inflated for ten minutes. Care should be taken for several hours after the block as postural hypotension may occur, particularly in elderly patients. Intravenous regional sympathetic block offers the advantage of being less invasive and uncomfortable for the patient than formal neural blockade. It provides blockade of sympathetic function for up to three days and occasionally longer. There is no modification of cholinergic activity.

Other drugs have been used with a similar technique as alternatives in circumstances where guanethidine is not available. These include reserpine, bretylium, prazocin and phentolamine.[15] Also tried by an intravenous regional technique have been clonidine, steroids, ketanserin, droperidol and numerous others.

There are almost no comparative studies of the treatment of sympathetic pain by nerve block. A comparative, randomized study found little difference between guanethidine block and formal sympathetic nerve block.[28] Another retrospective study reported better outcome with sympathetic block compared to more conservative measures.[29] Nearly all reported work concerns the success of a single treatment or technique, and thus falls into the category of self-fulfilling prophecy.

Somatic nerve blocks

There are arguments for trying somatic neural blockade if there is inadequate relief of pain following sympathetic block. Failure to respond to sympathetic blockade does not preclude a sympathetic pain, although some positive response to sympathetic blockade would be expected. Indeed, it may be that somatic blockade is necessary for the management of the established case as pain may be arising from somatic sources. Defalque reports a series where repeated axillary blocks were more effective than serial stellate ganglion blocks in the management of reflex sympathetic dystrophy.[30] There are numerous anecdotal reports of the value of somatic block in addition to sympathetic block in the management of advanced causalgia and reflex sympathetic dystrophy but no controlled studies.[31]

PHYSIOTHERAPY

There is widespread agreement that physiotherapy is a vital part of any treatment programme. The goal of therapy is to improve function and increase the range of movements in the painful area. Inevitably, this means that both passive and active assisted exercises are employed in combination with superficial heat, ultrasound and other therapy such as drugs and sympathetic blocks. The use of physiotherapy is non-specific, and usually, is not carried out under the direct supervision of the referring physician. There are no adequate comparative studies and it is rare for this treatment to be used alone. Frequently 'physiotherapy' is used as a generic term and one is left with the impression that no clear instructions accompany the patient to the physiotherapy department. It is rare for there to be mention of assessment, comparison of treatments, control groups or a rationale to the choice of one treatment or another.

There are reports that suggest that physiotherapy alone can be sufficient therapy for mild cases of sympathetic pain. Baker and Winegarner reported the successful treatment of 6 of 28 patients with physiotherapy.[32] They emphasized that early institution of treatment gave a greater chance of success, and they felt the physiotherapist should be both aggressive and enthusiastic. The reviews of Omer and Thomas[33] and Pak et al.[3] also report successful resolution of symptoms with physiotherapy alone. However, the nature of the successful physiotherapy varied and included elevation, traction, individual splints, exercising devices and something termed 'general body conditioning'. Lindblom has pointed out that the hyperalgesia found in reflex sympathetic dystrophy is not confined to mechanical stimuli and that patients may exhibit hyperalgesia to heat and/or cooling stimuli.[34] Thus, it is unsurprising that both cold and heat have been advocated as treatment.

The 'wet towel sign' is a well known presentation in which the patient wraps his or her affected extremity in a cold damp towel to try and obtain some symptomatic relief from the constant burning pain. Rather than being of benefit, it is more likely that hyperalgesia to cooling stimuli may characterize patients with sympathetic dystrophy. This has been demonstrated by Frost and her co-workers[35] who showed that patients with pain from mild cooling stimuli are likely to have a sympathetically-maintained component to their pain and may benefit from procedures directed at reducing sympathetic input into the painful area.

Heat is generally thought to be beneficial in the management of sympathetic pain. This can be applied in many forms, such as local heat by the use of lamps or baths, to diathermy and interferential therapy. The use of heat and cold for therapeutic purposes has been reviewed by Lehmann.[36]

STIMULATION PRODUCED ANALGESIA

Acupuncture

Electroacupuncture was used to treat successfully 14 of 20 patients with established sympathetic pain in one uncontrolled series.[37] All patients had received analgesics and physiotherapy for at least one month prior to treatment. The authors suggest that the decrease in pain associated with the electroacupuncture was responsible for the increased muscle power experienced by the majority of their patients. There was little or no improvement in range of movement in the affected limb.

Transcutaneous electrical nerve stimulation [TENS]

TENS has been used for some time to treat sympathetic pain, but published results are rare. The mechanism of action remains unclear although Meyer and Fields felt that selective large fibre activity was responsible for the clinical effect in their study of eight patients.[38] Two of the patients in this study were much better after treatment, 4 obtained transient relief and 2 were unchanged. TENS has been used to treat successfully sympathetic pain in adults and children.

Implanted peripheral nerve stimulators will be considered by Wells and Miles (this issue).

DRUG THERAPY

The apparently successful treatment of sympathetic pain by adrenergic blocking drugs, such as guanethidine given by intravenous regional technique, has prompted others to try many drugs in a similar fashion. Bretylium, reserpine, hydrallazine, thymoxamine, phenoxybenzamine, phentolamine, methyldopa, clonidine, naftidrofuryl, droperidol and even lysine acetylsalicylate have been used with varying degrees of success. Thus it would appear logical to try the systemic use of both alpha- and beta-adrenergic blocking drugs. Unfortunately, clinical trials of these drugs have met with limited success, despite several papers that claim outstanding results. This disappointing state of affairs probably reflects differences in the mechanisms of the many conditions that are known as reflex sympathetic dystrophy. However, there are reasonable grounds for believing that there may be a role for these agents in the management of sympathetic pain.

Alpha-adrenergic blocking drugs

Phenoxybenzamine is a postsynaptic α_1 and presynaptic α_2 blocking drug. Ghostine and co-workers reported an uncontrolled series of 40 patients successfully treated with increasing daily doses of 40 to 120 mg of this drug.[39] Duration of treatment was 6 to 8 weeks and total resolution of pain was achieved in all cases. Phentolamine has similar actions to phenoxybenzamine and has been used as treatment,[40] and also to predict the response to oral prazocin, a relatively selective α_1 adrenergic blocker.[41]

Beta-adrenergic blocking drugs

There are isolated case reports of the successful use of propranolol. The presumed mechanism is blockade of the pre-junctional β_2 receptor which will cause release of noradrenaline if stimulated.

Calcium-channel blocking drugs

Initial studies with these agents are in progress. In theory, these agents should have a beneficial effect as sympathomimetic amines depend upon calcium flux for their action. The alpha-adrenergic stimulation with noradrenaline produces peripheral vasoconstriction secondary to increased calcium entry and increased calcium mobilization in vascular smooth muscle cells. The β-adrenergic agonists augment the calcium influx by increasing the number of functional calcium channels. There are data which suggest that hypercalcaemia may stimulate both α- and β-adrenergic receptors although the results are variable.

Corticosteroids

There are early reports of the use of steroids in the management of shoulder hand syndrome and reflex sympathetic dystrophy.[42,43] These series are not controlled, but 82% of those patients who satisfied the diagnostic criteria for sympathetic pain had good or excellent responses to systemic corticosteroids. There was no relationship between the duration of symptoms and the clinical response, and many of the cases were of over 6 months duration.

A more recent paper employed a randomized, placebo-controlled design to study the effects of 30 mg of prednisone daily in divided doses. The study was continued until clinical resolution or 12 weeks. Improvement was seen in all the prednisone-treated patients at the end of the trial, with only 20% of the placebo group showing any improvement.[44] The mechanisms by which steroids help RSD are unclear. They may stabilize basement membranes and reduce capillary permeability, thereby decreasing the plasma extravasation associated with the early stages of the disease. However, this does not explain the apparent success of this sort of treatment in established cases.

Other drugs

There are reports of success with drugs as varied as the serotonin antagonist—ketanserin, non-steroidal anti-inflammatory drugs, neuroleptics (such as chlorpromazine and haloperidol), anti-depressives and anxiolytics, anticonvulsants, calcitonin and the enkephalinase inhibitor D-phenylalanine. None of the studies are controlled and many are little more than anecdotal.[45]

NEUROSURGERY

Tasker has reviewed the indications for the invasive treatment of sympathetic pain.[46] He states that the 'normal' invasive treatment for sympathetic pain usually consists of repeated sympathetic blocks or sensory blocks which may relieve the pain temporarily. He stresses that it is important to recognize that permanent surgical denervation at the same site as the block, usually fails to relieve the pain. He believes that such pain responds best to chronic stimulation, but notes that only 50% of apparently suitable candidates gain relief from stimulation, and that there is a tendency for patients to escape from control despite continued efficient operation of their stimulating device.

Experience with implanted peripheral nerve stimulators has been reported by Racz and his colleagues.[47] However, despite occasional reports of success with peripheral, epidural and 'central' stimulation, the overall picture remains gloomy and there seems to be little if any place for the use of destructive techniques in the management of sympathetic pain.

If the pain is arising from nerve damage, it seems unlikely that damaging some more nerves will be helpful.

BEHAVIOURAL ASPECTS

The need for the patient to take an active role in their own rehabilitation has been emphasized previously. It is important to provide support and encouragement for both patient and family during this period. If the disease process has become established it is easy to see how depression and anxiety may occur, as a natural response to a life of unrelieved pain. Both may require treatment in addition to the underlying pathological process. Assessment by either a psychiatrist or a psychologist should be considered if the disease process has existed for longer than six months.

MULTIDISCIPLINARY MANAGEMENT

Patients presenting with sympathetic pain may require the skills of many different members of the pain management team. The skills of the anaesthetists and physiotherapist are those most likely to be needed first. However, difficult or advanced cases may need assessment by other disciplines such as neurologists, neurosurgeons, pharmacologists, psychiatrists, psychologists and occupational therapists. No individual can know enough to be able to treat all aspects of chronic pain and multidisciplinary management represents the most likely method of achieving success.

SUMMARY

Successful treatment of sympathetic pain requires rapid assessment and appropriate therapy. Treatment should be directed at the restoration of normal function and can be achieved best with a combination of appropriate sympathetic or somatic nerve block in combination with physiotherapy. Other non-invasive therapy may be helpful.

REFERENCES

1 Abram SE, Blumberg H, Boas RA et al. Proposed definition of reflex sympathetic dystrophy. In: Stanton-Hicks M, Janig W, Boas RA, eds. Reflex sympathetic dystrophy. Boston: Kluwer, 1990: pp. 209–210
2 Abram SE. Reflex sympathetic dystrophy: Incidence and epidemiology. In: Stanton-Hicks M, Janig W, Boas RA, eds. Reflex sympathetic dystrophy. Boston: Kluwer, 1990: pp. 9–15
3 Pak TJ, Martin GM, Magness JL et al. Reflex sympathetic dystrophy. Minn Med 1970; 53: 507–512
4 Drucker WB, Hubay CA, Holden WD et al. Pathogenesis of post-traumatic sympathetic dystrophy. Am J Surg 1959; 97: 454–465
5 Carron H, Weller RW. Treatment of post-traumatic sympathetic dystrophy. In: Bonica JJ ed. Advances in Neurology, Vol 4. New York: Raven Press, 1974: pp. 485–490
6 Kleinert HE, Cole NM, Wayne L, et al. Post-traumatic sympathetic dystrophy. Orthop Clin North Am 1973; 4: 917–927
7 Rothberg JM, Tahmoush AJ, Oldakowski R. The epidemiology of causalgia among soldiers wounded in Vietnam. Milit Med 1983; 148: 347–350
8 Schwartzman RJ, McLellan TL. Reflex sympathetic dystrophy. A review. Arch Neurol 1987; 44: 555–561
9 Richards RL. Causalgia. A centennial review. Arch Neurol 1967; 16: 339–350

10 Echlin F, Owens FM, Wells WL. Observations of 'major' and 'minor' causalgia. J Nerv Ment Dis 1948; 107: 174–180

11 McQuay HJ, Carroll D, Moore RA. Postoperative orthopaedic pain—the effect of opiate premedication and local anaesthetic blocks. Pain 1988; 33: 291–296

12 Bach S, Noreng MF, Tjellden NU. Phantom limb pain in amputees during the first twelve months following limb amputation, after preoperative lumbar epidural blockade. Pain 1988; 33: 297–302

13 Wall PD. The prevention of postoperative pain. Pain 1988; 33: 289–290

14 Charlton JE. Current views on the use of nerve blocking in the relief of chronic pain. In: Swerdlow M ed. The therapy of pain. Lancaster: MTP Press, 1986: pp. 133–164

15 Lofstrom JB, Cousins MJ. Sympathetic neural blockade of upper and lower extremity. In: Cousins MJ, Bridenbaugh, PO eds. Neural blockade in clinical anesthesia and management of pain. 2nd edn. Philadelphia: Lippincott, 1988: pp. 461–500

16 Evans FJ. The placebo response in pain reduction. In: Bonica JJ, ed. Advances in neurology, Vol 4. New York: Raven Press, 1974: pp. 289–296

17 Arner S, Lindblom U, Meyerson BA, Molander C. Prolonged relief of neuralgia after regional anesthetic blocks. A call for further experimental and systematic clinical studies. Pain 1990; 43: 287–297

18 Wall PD. Neuropathic pain. Pain 1990; 43: 267–268

19 Boas RA. Sympathetic nerve blocks: their role in sympathetic pain. In: Stanton-Hicks M, Janig W, Boas RA, eds. Reflex sympathetic dystrophy. Boston: Kluwer, 1990: pp. 101–112

20 Scott DB. Techniques of regional anaesthesia. Norwalk: Appleton & Lange, 1989: pp. 206–209

21 Racz GB. Techniques of neurolysis. Boston: Kluwer, 1989: pp. 234–239

22 Winnie AP. An immobile needle for nerve blocks. Anesthesiology 1969; 31: 577–578

23 Hatangdi VS, Boas RA. Lumbar sympathectomy: A single needle technique. Br J Anaesth 1985; 57: 285–289

24 Boas RA, Hatangdi VS, Richards EG. Lumbar sympathectomy, a percutaneous chemical technique. In: Bonica JJ, Albe-Fessard D, eds. Advances in pain research and therapy, Vol 1. New York: Raven Press, 1976: pp. 685–689

25 Gregg RV, Constantin CH, Ford DJ, Raj PP, Means E. Electrophysiologic and histopathologic investigation of phenol in renographin as a neurolytic agent. Anesthesiology 1986; 63: A239

26 Hannington-Kiff JG. Intravenous regional sympathetic block with guanethidine. Lancet 1974; i: 1019–1021

27 Hannington-Kiff JG. Pharmacologic target blocks in painful dystrophic limbs. In: Wall PD, Melzack R, eds. Textbook of pain, 2nd edn. Edinburgh: Churchill Livingstone, 1989: pp. 754–766

28 Bonelli S, Conoscente F, Movilia PG, Restelli L, Francucci B, Grossi E. Regional intravenous guanethidine vs stellate ganglion block in reflex sympathetic dystrophies: A randomised trial. Pain 1983; 16: 297–307

29 Wang JK, Johnson KE, Istrup DM. Sympathetic blocks for reflex sympathetic dystrophy. Pain 1985; 23: 13–17

30 Defalque RJ. Axillary versus stellate ganglion blocks for reflex sympathetic dystrophy of the upper extremity. Regional Anesth 1984; 9: 35

31 Cicala RS, Jones JW, Westbrook LL. Causalgic pain responding to epidural but not to sympathetic nerve block. Anesth Analg 1990; 70: 218–219

32 Baker EG, Winegarner FG. Causalgia: a review of 28 treated cases. Am J Surg 1969; 117: 690–694

33 Omer G, Thomas S. Treatment of causalgia: review of cases at Brooke General Hospital. Texas Med 1971; 67: 63–67

34 Lindblom U. Neuralgia: mechanisms and therapeutic prospects. In: Benedetti

C. Chapman CR, Morrica G. eds. Advances in pain research and therapy, vol 7. New York: Raven Press, 1984: pp. 427–438

35 Frost SA, Raja SN, Campbell JN, Meyer RA, Khan AA. Does hyperalgesia to cooling stimuli characterize patients with sympathetically maintained pain (reflex sympathetic dystrophy)? In: Dubner R, Gebhart GF, Bond MR. eds. Proceedings of the Vth world congress on pain. Amsterdam: Elsevier, 1988: pp. 151–156

36 Lehman J. Therapeutic heat and cold. 4th edn. Baltimore: Williams and Wilkins, 1988

37 Chan CS, Chow SP. Electroacupuncture in the treatment of postramatic sympathetic dystrophy (Sudek's Atrophy). Br J Anaesth 1981; 53: 899–902

38 Meyer GA, Fields HL. Causalgia treated by selective large fibre stimulation of peripheral nerve. Brain 1972; 95: 163–168

39 Ghostine SY, et al. Phenoxybenzamine in the treatment of causalgia. J Neurosurg 1984; 60: 1263–1268

40 Campbell JN, Raja SN, Meyer RA. Painful sequelae of nerve injury. In: Dubner R, Gebhart GF, Bond MR. eds. Proceedings of the Vth world congress on pain. Amsterdam: Elsevier, 1988: pp. 135–143

41 Abram SE. Pain of sympathetic origin. In: Raj PP, ed. Practical management of pain. Chicago: Year Book Medical Publishers, 1986: pp. 451–463

42 Glick EN. Reflex dystrophy [algoneurodystrophy]. Results of treatment by corticosteroids. Rheumatol Rehab 1973; 12: 84–88

43 Kozin F, et al. The reflex sympathetic dystrophy syndrome. III. Scintigraphic studies, further evidence for the therapeutic activity of systemic corticosteroids, and proposed diagnostic criteria. Am J Med 1981; 70: 23–30

44 Christensen K, Jensen EM, Noer I. The reflex sympathetic dystrophy syndrome; response to treatment with systemic corticosteroids. Acta Chir Scand 1982; 148: 653–655

45 Charlton JE. Reflex sympathetic dystrophy; non-invasive methods of treatment. In: Stanton-Hicks M, Janig W, Boas RA, eds. Reflex sympathetic dystrophy. Boston: Kluwer, 1990: pp. 151–164

46 Tasker RR. Reflex sympathetic dystrophy—neurosurgical approaches. In: Stanton-Hicks M, Janig W, Boas RA. eds. Reflex sympathetic dystrophy. Boston: Kluwer, 1990: pp. 125–134

47 Racz GB, Lewis B Jr, Heavner JE, Scott J. Peripheral nerve stimulator implant for treatment of RSD. In: Stanton-Hicks M, Janig W, Boas RA, eds. Reflex sympathetic dystrophy. Boston: Kluwer, 1990: pp. 135–141

British Medical Bulletin (1991) Vol. 47, No. 3, pp. 619–630

Neuropathic pain and injured nerve: Peripheral mechanisms

M Devor
Neurobehavior Unit, Department of Zoology, Life Sciences Institute, Hebrew University of Jerusalem, Jerusalem, Israel

Injury to sensory axons often has the paradoxical effect of inducing positive sensory disturbances; paraesthesias and chronic neuropathic pain. Such symptoms can be at least partially understood in terms of pathophysiological changes that occur in the electrical excitability of the injured sensory neuron. These changes result in the generation of an abnormal ongoing and evoked discharge, originating, alternatively, at various ectopic neural pacemaker sites. Many of the most effective therapeutic modalities recommended for neuropathic pain act by reducing this ectopic neural discharge.

Injury or disease affecting peripheral nerves frequently triggers bizarre and intractible sensory abnormalities.[1] If a nerve is sectioned, the center of its peripheral innervation field is usually rendered unresponsive to applied stimuli. This anaesthesia, however, is often accompanied by a spontaneous feeling of numbness (swollen cheek, boxing-glove hands), and sometimes by disturbing paraesthesias and pain (anaesthesia dolorosa). Around the edges of the zone of anaesthesia, stimuli may evoke distorted, unnatural responses.

Partial injury may be even worse, triggering, in addition to ongoing pain, such neuropathic changes as intense pain to weak stimulation (allodynia), electric shock-like paroxysms, spread, delayed responses that build up to a painful crescendo, and reference to distant locations.

Together, these abnormalities constitute a theoretical challenge, and often a clinical nightmare. After all, block of nerve conduction, either complete or partial, ought to reduce sensation, not to increase it! This chapter on peripheral neuropathic processes, and the chapter by Wall on central ones (this issue), will attempt to outline a solution. Specifically, it will be shown that an injured nerve does not behave like a severed telephone cable, either letting through its message or not letting it through. Rather, nerve fibers undergo characteristic changes which result in the creation of false sensation, and the distortion of sensation elicited by applied stimuli. In general, abnormalities of neural processing develop in both the peripheral and the central nervous systems (PNS, CNS), even when the provoking injury is peripheral. Abnormal PNS responses are then processed by an abnormal CNS.[2]

ABNORMAL DISCHARGE IN INJURED NERVE FIBERS

Sensory axons in peripheral nerves are supported metabolically by the nerve cell body which resides in the (paraspinal) dorsal root ganglion (DRG). For this reason, when an axon has been severed, the portion distal to the injury degenerates, but the proximal stump survives. Experiments in laboratory animals, backed by neurographic observations in awake humans, have shown that the injured axons at the proximal stump, local patches of demyelination along the axon, and often the DRG cells as well, become sources of abnormal, ectopic discharge.[3-6] Abnormal impulses generated at these sites are conducted centrally into the spinal cord and brain, where they are interpreted as originating in the tissue (skin, muscle, viscera etc.) originally served by the intact nerve. The brain is generally unaware of the true ectopic source of the abnormal activity. This process can account for much of the ongoing sensory experience associated with nerve injury, both paraesthesias and neuropathic pain.

The cellular/molecular change responsible for the development of these foci of abnormal neural discharge is rapidly becoming clear. It appears to be related to the fact that the molecular constituents of nerve that are responsible for normal neural activity, particularly channel and receptor proteins, are synthesized in the cell body in the DRG, and transported anterogradely by rapid axoplasmic flow down the length of the axon toward the normal sensory ending. When the nerve is injured, the molecules simply dam up at the injury site (and perhaps also in the DRG cell).[7-9] Not subject to the regulatory processes that normally control the excitability of sensory endings, these sites are prone to becoming hyperexcitable, and hence sources of abnormal sensation and pain.

Structurally, the injured axon endings in peripheral nerves that generate ectopic neural discharge are minute (10–20 µm) swellings or axon 'endbulbs'. These may be massed within a small region of nerve (e.g. in a nerve end neuroma), or they may be disseminated throughout a nerve or its target tissue. They are not visible except using special histological procedures.[10,11] An example is shown in Figure 1. Because of their ability to generate repetitive firing independent of the normal sensory apparatus, they have been termed 'ectopic neural pacemaker nodules (or sites)'.

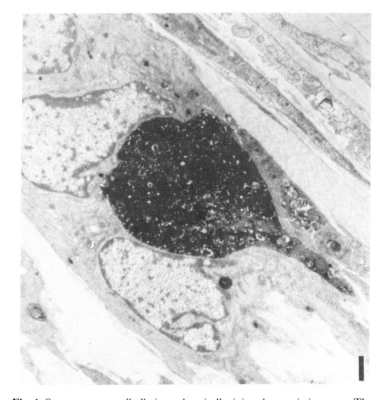

Fig. 1 Sensory axon endbulb in a chronically injured rat sciatic nerve. These structures, virtually invisible except when labelled using specialized procedures (anterograde transport of WGA-HRP in this case), are believed to be the structural counterpart of ectopic neural pacemaker nodules. Scale bar: 1 µm. (Image kindly provided by K. Fried. Details in Refs[8,10,11]).

ABNORMAL EVOKED RESPONSES

Ectopic neural pacemaker sites in injured nerve, in addition to firing spontaneously, become sensitive to a broad range of physical, chemical and metabolic challenges. For example, impulse activity is usually evoked at these sites by mechanical stimulation. This accounts for the well-known Tinel sign, evoked by tapping along the course of an affected nerve. Less well appreciated is the prominent mechanosensitivity of DRGs and injured dorsal roots. Mechanical stresses often impinge on these structures when there is vertebral column involvement, or when a nerve trunk is stretched as in the Lasegue sign (pain on straight leg raising).

Sites of potential nerve constriction (e.g. the carpal tunnel), or transit points of small branches across fascial planes are locations of special risk. Conditions here are ripe both for the production of ectopic neural pacemaker nodules upon local trauma, and *also* for their mechanical stimulation during body movement. Although unproved, the characteristic ache of myofascial pain, and its associated local trigger points, suggests an origin in ectopic neural pacemaker nodules formed where, for example, dorsal rami cross into paraspinal muscles of the lower back.

Ectopic neural pacemaker sites display other significant sensitivities too.[3-5] They are powerfully excited by ischemia and anoxia, they are aroused by certain inflammatory mediators, and many (C-fibers) are paradoxically excited by cold.[12] This latter sensitivity may account for cold intolerance (e.g. in some amputees).

An unexpected sensitivity of ectopic neural pacemaker sites is to circulating and locally released catecholamines. This is believed to be the basis for pain in causalgia and related reflex sympathetic dystrophies (RSD), and for the fact that these pains are frequently relieved by sympathectomy.[3-5,12]

Abnormal discharge may be evoked or exacerbated by any combination of these factors and others. Thus, removal of any single one (e.g. by sympathectomy) will not necessarily relieve the pain.

ENDOGENOUS RHYTHMICITY OF ECTOPIC NEURAL PACEMAKER SITES

Action potential discharge in afferents innervating skin, muscle, viscera etc. is under the second-to-second control of sensory receptor endings (generator potential). For this reason normal sensation is tightly coupled in time, space, and modality (sensory quality) to the stimulus. Ectopic neural pacemaker sites in affected nerves and DRGs are different as they are capable of autonomous firing.[4,5] Consequently once triggered, by a brief mechanical stimulus, for example, they may continue to fire for seconds, minutes or even hours (Fig. 2). Such behaviour is a likely explanation of neuro-pathic aftersensation.

Following particularly intense bursts of such abnormal activity, ectopic pacemaker sites typically become refractory for a period of time, so that subsequent stimuli are temporarily ineffective in gen-erating bursts.[4,5] Such post-attack refractoriness is typical of cer-tain clinical neuralgias (e.g. trigeminal neuralgia).[1]

In experimental preparations, most ectopic pacemakers appear to be poised close to their 'threshold for endogenous rhythmic firing'. Some have ongoing discharge at rest. Others, usually silent,

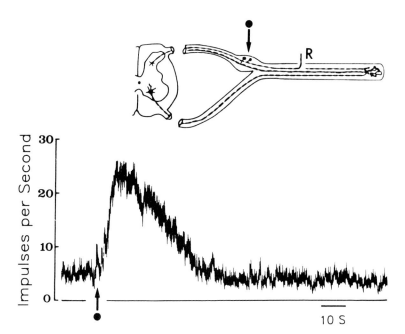

Fig. 2 Afterdischarge at an ectopic neural pacemaker site in a rat whose sciatic nerve was injured 11 days previously. In this experiment, spontaneous discharge (ca. 5 impulses per second), originating in the 5th lumbar DRG, was recorded at electrode R. Momentary application to the ganglion of a weak force (arrow, 150 mg for 0.5 s) caused a burst of activity reaching 5 × the baseline firing rate, and lasting for about a minute. Similar, often more prolonged responses can be evoked from ectopic neural pacemaker nodules in chronic injured nerves.

may issue massive bursts of action potential discharge when nudged ever so slightly by a mechanical or other stimulus. This hairtrigger characteristic is presumably responsible for the paroxysmal nature of some neuropathic pains.

'Threshold straddling' by ectopic neural pacemaker nodules holds out possible opportunities for treatment. Because of it, a relatively subtle suppression of excitability (by membrane stabilization, for example), is potentially capable of having profound and selective effects on neuropathic pain. That is, for ectopic impulse generating sites just above threshold for repetitive firing, low doses of appropriate drugs can switch the site from ongoing firing at substantial rates to complete silence. This effect need not interfere with impulse generation and propagation in neighbouring healthy axons.[14]

CROSS-EXCITATION AMONG ECTOPIC NEURAL PACEMAKER SITES

Normal sensory axons are highly isolated impulse conduction channels. Activity in one fiber has essentially no effect on the activity of neighbours. Injured or diseased neurons, in contrast, show several abnormal forms of cross-excitation. This is due to two related factors: (1) the basic hyperexcitability of ectopic neural pacemaker sites, and (2) the disruption of glial ensheathment of the individual neurons. One example of cross-excitation has been already mentioned: the pathophysiological coupling of (efferent) sympathetic and (afferent) sensory axons in RSD. This is an example of aberrant **chemical** crosstalk. Here, noradrenaline (and perhaps also peptide mediators) released from sympathetic neurons excites sensory neurons, abnormally adrenosensitive because of the injury, resulting in pain (*see* McMahon, this issue).[3−5,13]

Another type of cross-excitation depends on direct electrical coupling of axons (ephaptic crosstalk). Here, impulse activity in one sensory (or motor) axon drives impulse activity in a second.[15,16] It has been proposed recently that explosive activity triggered by ephaptic crosstalk accounts for pain in hemifacial spasm, some referred sensations, and perhaps even trigeminal neuralgia.[15−18]

A third type of cross-excitation that is of potential importance for understanding clinical symptomatology is 'crossed afterdischarge'. In this phenomenon, unlike ephaptic crosstalk, impulses are not coupled in a tight one-to-one manner. Rather, the activity of a group of neurons asynchronously engages the endogenous, repetitive firing capability of their neighbours.[19-21] It is still not clear whether this type of coupling is mediated by chemical neurotransmitters (as is sympathetic-sensory coupling), or by an alternative mechanism such as the gradual accumulation of K^+ ions in the extracellular space.

Crossed afterdischarge has been demonstrated both at nerve injury sites and in DRGs. The latter ectopic neural pacemaker site is particularly significant as it has the potential of accounting for much of the abnormal sensibility seen after partial nerve injuries. Consider the experiment illustrated in Figure 3. Many of the sensory neurons in the L4 and L5 DRGs in this animal were firing spontaneously, at least in part because of a partial injury of the sciatic nerve. The discharge of one such cell is shown. During the period indicated, impulse activity was evoked in neighbouring intact axons simply by rubbing the skin of the foot which was still partially innervated. As can be seen, this activity in neighbours substantially **increased** the ongoing activity of the axon under study, even though its own peripheral axon was cut so that it could not be stimulated directly from the skin. Cross-excitation in this case occured in the DRG.[21]

VARIABILITY

Perhaps the most puzzling feature of neuropathic pain states is their tremendous variability from time to time, place to place, and particularly, from individual to individual. The fact that a specific, well defined injury (e.g. below the knee amputation), can cause crippling pain in one patient and none at all in another, frequently raises the suspicion of hidden agendas. However, notwithstanding the reality of psychosocial variables in the expression of pain behaviour, there are sound **neurophysiological** reasons for the variability of symptoms according to the ectopic neural pacemaker hypothesis.

The first has to do with variability in the initial formation of ectopic neural pacemaker sites. Animal experiments show that different nerves, and different sensory axon types, respond differentially to injury.[4] Furthermore, the response is dynamic in time. In rat sciatic nerve A-axons, for example, neural activity originating at injury sites in peripheral nerve or dorsal root is high during the first 2–3 weeks post-operative, and then subsequently declines.[4,22] Activity in C-fibers is different, increasing more

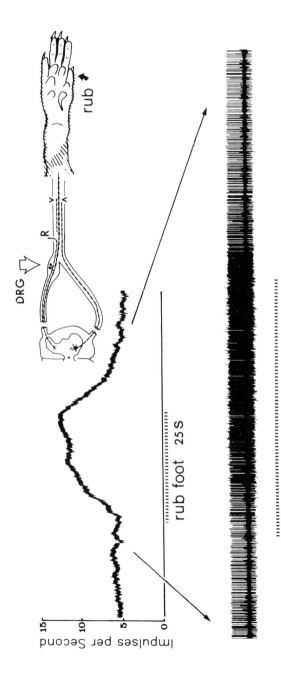

Fig. 3 Cross-excitation in a DRG after partial injury of the sciatic nerve in a rat. (*See text* for explanation, and Ref.[21] for further details).

slowly, and then remaining elevated for an extended period of time. The location at which a particular axon is injured may also be important.[22] These types of variability are dependent on intrinsic and extrinsic factors responsible for the initial **formation** of ectopic neural pacemaker sites.

A second type of variability has to do with those stimuli which **activate** ectopic neural pacemaker sites that have already formed. As noted above, such sites may be silent, or at least relatively silent, until activated by mechanical, thermal, chemical stimuli or metabolic events. For example, a region of potential abnormal impulse initiation may not become symptomatic until local adhesions, or a change in posture, causes undue mechanical forces to be brought to bear. Similarly, events (stress?) that elevate local sympathetic tone may exacerbate symptoms.[1]

Finally, there appear to be idiosyncratic, inherent individual differences in the likelihood that ectopic neural discharge will develop after injury. Ectopic neural activity differs quantitatively among species of experimental animals, and even among genetic strains of a particular species.[4] Recent evidence, based on a behavioural model of anaesthesia dolorosa (autotomy), strongly suggests that the propensity to develop neuropathic pain symptoms is inherited.[23] Indeed, a single recessive gene appears to be involved, in the rat model, at least. Needless to say, identification of the gene product is of substantial interest.

IMPLICATIONS FOR TREATMENT

A variety of current treatment approaches are targeted at peripheral sites of abnormal impulse discharge rather than the CNS. The most straightforward is blockage of the propagation of ectopic impulses into the CNS. This is readily accomplished by peripheral nerve, plexus, or epidural block using local anaesthetics. The main practical limitations are lack of selectivity (normal sensation and motor control are blocked too), and the relatively short duration of action of all available local anaesthetics. Note that when nerve or plexus block is ineffective, an ectopic source in DRGs needs to be considered before it can be concluded that the pain symptoms originate in the CNS.

Neurectomy, which should permanently block impulse propagation, is often only transiently effective. The reason is presumably re-formation of ectopic neural pacemaker sites. Dorsal rhizotomy ought to solve this problem. However, rhizotomy causes massive degeneration of central (spinal) terminals and hence true deafferentation pain.

A second approach is to remove stimuli which exacerbate ectopic neural discharge. Padding prostheses, mobilization of nerve ends into soft tissue, or otherwise protecting mechanosensitive sites are simple examples. Chemical or surgical sympatholysis, and local temperature regulation, are two others (see Charlton, this issue).

A third, and more sophisticated approach, is to relieve the underlying hyperexcitability of ectopic neural pacemaker sites by membrane stabilization. This is probably the mechanism of analgesia effected using systemic local anaesthetics.[24] Since the repetitive firing process is much more sensitive to these agents than is impulse conduction along the length of the nerve[14], abnormal firing, and hence abnormal pain sensation, may be reduced selectively.[24] Likewise, this factor may account for reports of pain relief following local nerve block that outlast the conduction blocking action of the local anaesthetic. The low residual drug levels remaining in the tissue, or in the circulation, may well be sufficient to hold ectopic pacemaker sites below their threshold for repetitive firing despite the fact that they are insufficient to stop the propagation of nerve impulses already generated.

There are several strategies for achieving membrane stabilization for extended periods of time. One example is the use of systemic anticonvulsants (e.g. phenytoin [Dilantin], or carbamazepine [Tegretol]). It has long been presumed that these act by reducing seizure-like activity in the CNS.[25] However, the recent demonstration of a dramatic suppressive action of phenytoin and carbamazepine on ectopic neural pacemaker sites in the PNS[26,27] requires that this presumption be re-evaluated. One practical limitation to the systemic use of both local anaesthetics and anticonvulsants is the fact that currently available preparations all pass the blood brain barrier and enter the brain. CNS depressant effects limit the doses that can be achieved in peripheral tissues.

An additional approach of this type involves the use of locally administered corticosteroids.[28] In addition to their anti-inflammatory actions, corticosteroids are membrane stabilizers, and are thus effective in suppressing ectopic neural pacemaker activity.[29] Unlike local anaesthetics, however, they are available in slow-release (depot) form that persists for several weeks. The stabilization of ectopic neural pacemaker nodules may be the main mode of action of corticosteroids when injected into painful trigger-points.

Finally, since the creation of ectopic neural pacemaker sites appears to be dependent on axoplasmic transport, it has been suggested that transport block using intra- or perineural application of one of the well known antimitotic agents (e.g. colchicine, vinblastin) might prove to be a useful treatment strategy.[30]

PERSPECTIVE

Nerve injury and disease triggers the creation in the nerve of minute neural pacemaker nodules, and augments abnormal discharge from sensory cell bodies in the affected DRGs. The abnormal firing characteristics of these ectopic impulse generating sites can account for much of the bizarre symptomatology associated with neuropathic pain states. Many current treatment modalities act by blocking or controlling ectopic neural activity, and new, still more effective drugs could presumably be designed with this aim in mind.

ACKNOWLEDGEMENTS

Supported by grants from the United States-Israel Binational Science Foundation (BSF), and the German-Israel Foundation for Scientific Research (GIF).

REFERENCES

1 Sunderland S. Nerves and nerve injuries. London: Churchill-Livingston, 1978
2 Devor M, Basbaum AI, Bennett GJ et al. Mechanisms of neuropathic pain following peripheral injury. In: Basbaum AI, Besson JM, eds. Towards a new pharmacotherapy of pain. Dahlem Konferenzen, London: Wiley 1990
3 Wall PD, Gutnick M. Ongoing activity in peripheral nerves: the physiology and pharmacology of impulses originating from a neuroma. Exp Neurol 1974; 43: 580–593
4 Devor M. The pathophysiology of damaged peripheral nerves. In: Wall PD, Melzack R, eds. Textbook of pain 2nd edition. London: Churchill-Livingston, 1989: pp. 63–81
5 Devor M, Rappaport ZH. Pain and the pathophysiology of damaged nerve. In: Fields H, ed. Pain syndromes in neurology. London: Butterworths, 1990: pp. 47–81
6 Nordin M, Nystrom B., Wallin U, Hagbarth K-E. Ectopic sensory discharges and paraesthesias in patients with disorders of peripheral nerves, dorsal roots, and dorsal columns. Pain 1984; 20: 231–245
7 Laduron PM. Axonal transport of presynaptic receptors. In: Smith RS, Bisby M. eds. Axonal transport. New York: Liss 1987. pp. 347–363
8 Devor M, Keller CH, Deerinck TJ, Levinson SR, Ellisman MH. Na$^+$ channel accumulation on axolemma of afferent endings in nerve end neuromas in *Apteronotus*. Neurosci Lett 1989; 102: 149–154

9 Brismar T, Gilly Wm F. Synthesis of sodium channels in the cell bodies of squid giant axons. Proc Nat Acad Sci 1987; 84: 1459–1463
10 Fried K, Devor M. End-structure of afferent axons injured in the peripheral and central nervous system. Somatosens. Motor Res 1988; 6: 79–99
11 Fried K, Govrin-Lippmann R, Rosenthal F, Ellisman MH, Devor M. Ultrastructure of afferent axon endings in a neuroma. J Neurocytol 1991, in press
12 Matzner O, Devor M. Contrasting thermal sensitivity of spontaneously active A- and C-fibers in experimental nerve-end neuromas. Pain 1987; 30: 373–384
13 Devor M, Janig W. Activation of myelinated afferents ending in a neuroma by stimulation of the sympathetic supply in the rat. Neurosci Lett 1981; 24: 43–47
14 Matzner O, Devor M. Sodium ion electrogenesis in nerve end neuroma. Eur J Neurosci 1988; (Suppl. 1): 173
15 Rasminsky M. Ephaptic transmission between single nerve fibres in the spinal nerve roots of dystrophic mice. J Physiol 1980; 305: 151–169
16 Seltzer Z, Devor M. Ephaptic transmission in chronically damaged peripheral nerves. Neurology 1979; 29: 1061–1064
17 Nielsen VK. Pathophysiology of hemifacial spasm: I. Ephaptic transmission and ectopic excitation. Neurology 1984; 34: 418–426
18 Raymond SA, Rocco AG. Ephaptic coupling of large fibers as a clue to mechanism in chronic neuropathic allodynia following damage to dorsal roots. Pain 1990; suppl. 5: 523
19 Lisney SJW, Devor M. Afterdischarge and interactions among fibers in damaged peripheral nerve in the rat. Brain Res 1987; 415: 122–136
20 Devor M, Dubner R. Centrifugal activity in afferent C-fibers influences the spontaneous afferent barrage generated in nerve-end neuromas. Brain Res 1988; 446: 396–400
21 Devor M, Wall PD. Cross-excitation in dorsal root ganglia of nerve injured and intact rats. J Neurophysiol 1990; 64: 1733–1746
22 Papir-Kricheli D, Devor M. Abnormal impulse discharge in primary afferent axons injured in the peripheral versus the central nervous system. Somatosens. Motor Res 1988; 6: 63–77
23 Devor M, Raber P. Heritability of symptoms in an experimental model of neuropathic pain. Pain 1990; 42: 51–67
24 Boas RA, Covino BG, Shahnarian A. Analgesic responses to IV lidocaine. Br J Anaesth 1982; 54: 501–505
25 Swerdlow M. Review: anticonvulsant drugs and chronic pain. Clin Neuropharm 1984; 7: 51–82
26 Yaari Y, Devor M. Phenytoin suppresses spontaneous ectopic discharge in rat sciatic nerve neuromas. Neurosci Lett 1985; 58: 117–122
27 Burchiel KJ. Carbemazepine inhibits spontaneous activity in experimental neuromas. Exp Neurol 1988; 102: 249–253
28 Travell JG, Simons DG. Myofascial pain and dysfunction: the trigger point manual. Baltimore: Williams and Wilkins, 1984
29 Devor M, Govrin-Lippmann R, Raber P. Corticosteroids suppress ectopic neuronal discharge originating in experimental neuromas. Pain 1985; 22: 127–137
30 Devor M, Govrin-Lippmann R. Axoplasmic transport block reduces ectopic impulse generation in injured peripheral nerves. Pain 1983; 16: 73–85

British Medical Bulletin (1991) Vol. 47, No. 3, pp. 631–643
© The British Council 1991

Neuropathic pain and injured nerve: Central mechanisms

P D Wall
Department of Anatomy & Developmental Biology, University College London, London, UK

A satisfactory explanation of neuropathic pain must include mechanisms capable of generating three types of pain: ongoing, episodic and allodynic. It must explain why many such pains develop very soon after injury while others occur after long delays. It must take into account the many painless neuropathies and the unpredictable relationship of the pain to the pathology in the painful neuropathies. While these diseases clearly start in the periphery and peripheral changes must contribute to the pain, there are also three types of central change. First changes in the afferent impulse barrage can induce long term shifts of central synaptic excitability. Second, changes of the chemical substances transported from the periphery to the cord produce alterations of cord cell excitability. Third, central control mechanisms can change into a pathological state permitting hyperexcitability. The combined peripheral and central pathology offers more than explanation since each factor could be a target for prevention as well as cure.

If the classical specificity theory of pain mechanisms was correct, this chapter would be very short because there are no relevant central mechanisms in that scheme. Classically the sensation of pain was considered as being created by the presence of nerve impulses in nociceptors which are conducted to the spinal cord over specialized fibres which excite nociceptive specific cells which in turn project to the pain centre by way of the spinothalamic tract. Since these central mechanisms were considered no more than a reliable transmission relay system, central mechanisms were simple slaves to the information generated in peripheral nerve fibres. If patients were sufficiently injudicious as to report painful sensations which appeared not to match the activity of peripheral nerves they were assigned to a mental limbo reserved for neurotics, hypochondriacs, or hallucinators. The specificity theory is not correct however and it is now widely appreciated that central mechanisms contribute to the painful consequences of diseases which are clearly initially limited to the periphery.

In considering the origin of these pains in a more subtle way than implied by the classical specificity theory, it will be necessary to move beyond the presence or absence of pain. Neuropathic pains have six characteristics which require an explanation in the periphery or in the central nervous system or by a combination of both. The characteristics of neuropathic pains are:

1. Some pains are ongoing and little influenced by peripheral stimuli.
2. Some pains are lancinating spontaneous stabs.
3. Some pains are provoked by normally innocuous stimuli (allodynia).
4. All pains except trigeminal neuralgia are associated with hypaesthesia.
5. Provoked pains require summation by prolongation, movement and repetition of the stimulus.
6. Provoked pains frequently demonstrate a delay and build up after the beginning of the stimulus.
7. Some pain states appear immediately after nerve injury, others after delays.

All seven of these characteristics could be used to indicate the likely existence of an abnormal central component in the pain. Devor, in the preceding chapter, has described the nature of ectopic sources of impulses which appear in damaged nerve. Each example which he has given of a source of ongoing activity is accompanied by an increase of mechanical sensitivity. Therefore one would expect to be able to locate the peripheral source of an ongoing pain by mechanical probing, the Tinel sign. This is frequently not apparent. In postherpetic neuralgia, for example where allodynia has not appeared or has been alleviated by TENS or sympathectomy, a deep ongoing pain which is not exaggerated by palpation is frequently present. Patients with postherpetic neuralgia show a mixture of three sensory signs, allodynia, anaes-

NEUROPATHIC PAIN AND INJURED NERVE: CENTRAL MECHANISMS   633

thesia and ongoing deep pain. The latter is the particular characteristic of patients with brachial plexus avulsions where their lesion lies in roots central to the dorsal root ganglia. The pain of such patients can only have a central origin since the input from the periphery has been entirely destroyed. The storms of lancinating stabs of pain from which many amputees suffer can similarly not be easily attributed to the periphery since they can rarely be provoked and no reports exist of such synchronous outbursts in animal model ectopic sources. The obvious explanation for allodynia is that the disease has sensitized previously high threshold peripheral fibres. However, as reviewed by Campbell et al.,[1] much recent research points to a central component in which normal low threshold sensory afferents excite hyperexcitable spinal cord cells as described by Woolf (this issue). The most obvious examples of pain produced by gentle stimulation of normal afferents are the allodynic areas always found on the stumps of amputees at a distance from the area of damage created by the injury or the surgery.[2] The next three characteristics, hypaesthesia with allodynia associated with summation and delay were first emphasized by Noordenbos.[3] Here pain is frequently not evoked by a single brief innocuous stimulus. However, if a light mechanical stimulus is repeated or a mild thermal stimulus is maintained, the patient often escalates from no response to feeling a minor sensation to excrutiating pain taking tens of seconds to reach maximum quite unlike normal responses. As he pointed out, it would be extremely difficult to explain this syndrome by pathological peripheral characteristics and he proposed central disinhibition as a likely alternative. Finally a severe limitation on possible mechanisms is provided by the observation that neuropathic pain states may have an extremely rapid onset. Obviously in certain painful neuropathies where the disease is of insidious onset such as diabetes or alcoholic neuropathies, it is not possible to identify the time of disease onset and of pain onset. However, accidental or surgical nerve damage is frequently followed by a very rapid and abrupt onset of severe pain often apparent after amputation or thoracotomy as the patient recovers from the anaesthetic.[4] It is true that there is a subsequent slow evolution of the nature and distribution of the pain but since the major problem is immediately apparent and since no animal models of peripheral change have such rapid onset, our attention is again directed to possible central explanations.

    In addition to incorporating the nature of the symptomatology in any satisfactory explanation, it is equally necessary to include an explanation of the absence of pain in certain nerve lesions such as:

Analgesic polyneuropathy[5]
Tangier disease[6]
Friedrich's ataxia[7]
Chronic renal failure[8]
Crush lesions[9]

A possible explanation for the first three is that they are in fact congenital disorders and that their tendency to produce pain by deafferentation may be overwhelmed by the restorative abilities of the developing nervous system. The absence of pain in the massive destruction of peripheral nerves in uraemic patients may be excused by the obvious existence of a general systemic disorder which could, without any evidence, prohibit the development of hyperexcitable tissue either in the periphery or centrally. The lack of pain following crush lesions of peripheral nerves is agreed by all, with such patients suffering paraesthesias at worst. Clearly this fact must be incorporated in any satisfactory explanation. Perhaps the most surprising pain free neuropathy is so common that it is never mentioned, tooth extraction. Here a branch of the fifth nerve is crudely avulsed and left to lie untended in the debris of the frequently infected tooth socket. Obviously chronic complaints must be very rare indeed or this procedure would not have persisted with such abandon over the centuries. Only rare or very rare or non-sequitur sequalae are mentioned, phantom tooth pain[10] dry socket syndrome, a possible causalgia like phenomenon normally attributed to infection[11] and atypical facial neuralgia.[12] Many assign the latter diagnosis to a psychiatric category as is apparent by such sentences as 'almost all are young women with significant psychopathology'.[13] The evident absence of chronic pain in the vast majority of those who suffer tooth extraction is particularly surprising since the trigeminal system has a highly specific form of painful fragility which results in trigeminal neuralgia, a condition which has no equivalent in other segments of the body. Furthermore 15% of cases of postherpetic neuralgia suffer pain in the trigeminal area and facial trauma with nerve damage may result in chronic neuropathic pain.

Clearly the existence of pain free neuropathies as well as painful ones should provide a clue as to the mechanism of the pain. In addition we are faced with a similar challenging fact that chronic pain is never present in 100% of the cases with the pathology to which the pain is commonly attributed. This variable relation of pathology with pain is not a monopoly of neuropathies since it plagues an understanding of the pain in much more common diseases such as cardiac ischaemia and osteoarthritis. Amputation is an example of major nerve damage with painful consequences occurring with great severity in only a fraction of the cases.[14] In our series of military casualties seen within months of their injury and again 10–15 years later, 67% were in the same pain on both occasions.[2] These fractions are explained away without evidence as attributable either to the variations in the nature of the lesion or more commonly are attributed to central factors particularly attitude.[15] The variation of the peripheral damage cannot be so easily used as an explanation where the results of the same surgeons' elective leg amputations were examined after 6 and 12 months with 50% of the patients in severe pain.[16] If the cause was the precise nature of the nerve lesions then either none or all of these patients should have been in pain. A genetic predisposition is proposed as a possible explanation based on the demonstration of a single recessive gene involved in the reaction of rats to sciatic section.[17] However, I have urged great caution in the premature attribution of single peripheral or central factors as the explanation of the puzzling variability of the relation of pain to nerve damage.[18] A major reason for this caution is a study of patients with intractable chronic causalgia following partial nerve lesions.[19] These patients had the site of the original partial nerve damage reconstructed by total nerve resection of the damaged area followed by cable grafting of the sural nerve across the gap of the excised nerve. All patients successfully regenerated their nerves across the graft but relapsed into the precise state and location of the pain they had experienced before the graft. The relevance of that finding to this chapter is two fold. These patients were not peculiarly susceptible to nerve lesions since the sural lesions produced no sequelae. Second since the surgeons cut the entire nerve but the symptoms recurred only in that fraction of the nerves' territory involved in the original trauma, there must have been something special about that incident which originated from those particular damaged nerves, but was maintained even when the original area of damage was excised. This observation among many drives one to seek some mechanism initiated by local damage but located central to the lesion.

In seeking peripheral and central mechanisms responsible for

neuropathic pain, we must incorporate mechanisms that are capable of generating:
A. Three types of pain: (1) ongoing; (2) episodic; and (3) provoked with the spatial and temporal characteristics of allodynia.
B. Pains associated with some types of nerve lesion and not with others.
C. Pains associated with only a fraction of apparently identical lesions.

Three quite separate classes of central mechanism must be considered:
1. Central changes generated by arriving nerve impulses or their absence.
2. Central changes generated by substances transported from the periphery or their absence.
3. Central changes generated by instability of central control mechanisms.

Just as central and peripheral explanations are not contradictory and mutually exclusive these three different central mechanisms could all be operative. It is to be hoped that one mechanism will predominate in a particular patient at a particular time since therapy would thereby be easier.

AFFERENT IMPULSE INDUCED CENTRAL CHANGES

Impulse triggered central hyperexcitability

We now know, thanks to the work of Woolf and his collaborators as described in this issue, that an afferent barrage, particularly in the unmyelinated afferents originating from deep tissue, triggers a long lasting change of the excitability of dorsal horn cells. This increased excitability is provoked by the arriving impulses but maintained by central mechanisms. It may be that the trigger is the emission of peptides from the terminals of unmyelinated afferents. The brief input is followed by a series of prolonged alterations in the dorsal horn cells in which the membrane and chemistry of the cells change. These changes are now the subject of widespread research including the manipulation of NMDA receptors, and activity and calcium dependent changes of enzyme activity within the cell. The onset of such changes is strongly influenced by NMDA receptor blockers and by narcotics. The latency of onset occurs within seconds to minutes of the arriving barrage. They are therefore candidates for explaining the rapidity of onset of some of the pains with which we are concerned. The duration of these central changes after an abrupt brief input volley has so far been shown in animal models to last for hours. In order to explain chronic pains triggered by a brief episode, it would be necessary to demonstrate persistance of central hyperexcitability for which there is so far no evidence. However, the animal experimental test inputs and the observation periods have been restricted in time and intensity. It is possible that the observed changes may themselves set off more fundamental and irreversible changes in the cells and this is now being investigated. It is also possible that once triggered by an initial large input, the prolonged changes might be maintained by a trickle of abnormal afferent inputs. This would result in an abnormal central component maintained in part by a continuous low level of pathological peripheral input.

If the classical picture of dorsal horn pain mechanisms was true, an increase of excitability would not explain the origin of the symptoms which interest us here. If pain was only to be attributed to the firing of nociceptive specific cells, an increase of their excitability would produce only hyperalgesia, that is to say an increase of the amount of pain produced by normally painful stimuli and would not produce allodynia. However, these nociceptive specific cells are the minority of the cells which signal noxious events in the periphery. By far the commonest cells respond not only to injury but also to gentle stimuli and are called convergent or wide dynamic range cells.[20-22] In comparing the onset of aversive behaviour in monkeys with the onset of firing of convergent versus nociceptive specific cells, it appears that 'pain behaviour' is best related to the response of the convergent cells.[23] Furthermore, Cook et al.,[24] showed that under conditions of afferent induced central hyperexcitability, nociceptive specific cells could convert to the convergent variety. Taken together these results support the suggestion that a hyperexcitable response of such cells could be responsible for the allodynic aspects of neuropathic pain where normally innocuous stimuli provoke pain. Furthermore, since these cells gradually increase their output with repeated inputs, the 'wind up' phenomenon,[25] they could be the arbitrators of the temporal and spatial summation which is a critical feature of the pain evoked in the patients we consider here. As the excitability of central cells rises so does their ongoing activity. Therefore a sufficient increase of excitability produced by the mechanism discussed here and by others to be discussed could result in a high enough level of ongoing activity to form the basis of the continuous ongoing pains.

Impulse triggered central degeneration

The basis of this possible mechanism depends on the extensive work of Sugimoto most recently reported in Sugimoto et al.[26] When nerves are cut a brief maximal frequency volley is generated in all types of afferents, the injury discharge. It is probable that in normal spinal cord, there are limiting mechanisms which prevent the postsynaptic arrival of such massive volleys. These depend partly on the impulse carrying ability of the terminal arborizations of afferents and partly on the presence of inhibitory mechanisms, both of which limit the maximal effective size of inputs. Sugimoto's original observations showed that central cells degenerated following section of trigeminal afferents if the inhibitory mechanisms had been disabled by strychnine. Now it has been observed that such degenerating neurons occur in the dorsal horn without strychnine but in the presence of a particularly evocative partial nerve lesion in rats developed by Bennett & Xie.[27] This partial nerve lesion produced by constriction results in a very prolonged hyperpathic state. It is accompanied by a massive ongoing afferent barrage originating from the dorsal root ganglia presumably by the mechanism described in the chapter by Devor (this issue). Furthermore, it is likely that such a lesion may simultaneously abolish the normal presynaptic and postsynaptic inhibitions in dorsal horn as was shown to occur after sciatic lesions.[28,29] Therefore a combination of increased afferent barrage with decreased central inhibition may permit such a catastrophic increase of synaptic excitation that cells die by the now well established mechanism of amino acid excitotoxicity. It could be that this effect is the extreme end result of Woolf's hyperexcitability process described in the section above. Induced degeneration would be one way in which temporary hyperexcitability could be converted to permanent and irreversible changes.

The absence of afferent impulses

Arriving sensory impulses over dorsal roots to the dorsal horn produce both excitations and inhibitions. A reduction of sensory input therefore may reduce both. This would result in a partial disinhibition which is presumably the explanation for the immediate appearance of a phantom limb after plexus local anaesthesia.[30] Local anaesthesia of peripheral nerves or epidurally or intrathecally frequently unmasks pain in addition to the expected anaesthesia.[31] Partial blockade was the basis of Noordenbos'[3] theory of hyperpathic states. Some support is provided by the success of stimulation in normalizing sensation after partial nerve injuries[32] and of TENS[33] where the intention is to generate an afferent barrage which has been prevented by the disease. This section is introduced to emphasize the fact that pain may be the consequence of an increase of excitation or of a decrease of inhibition.

CENTRAL CHANGES INDUCED BY CHEMICAL TRANSPORT

All nerve cells transport crucial chemicals for their survival from the cell body to the far reaches of the cell and back from a distance to the cell body. If an axon is cut in the periphery, the dorsal root ganglia change chemically, physiologically and pharmacologically as a consequence of the changed transport.[34,35] Interruption of impulse traffic alone does not produce these changes.[36] They are produced by a failure of normal transport of substances, such as nerve growth factor,[37] or by the leaking in of foreign substances in the area of damage. Crushing a nerve does not produce nearly such severe changes as cutting the nerve[38] an observation which is clearly evocative of the paradox that nerve section has much more severe pain sequelae than crushing the nerve. The explanation for this difference may be that the sprouts which grow from crushed axons are rapidly in contact with Schwann cells which provide a substitute supply of nerve growth factor whereas in the neuroma sprouts growing from cut axons contact many unusual cells. After the cutting of axons and the failure of regeneration, the changes in dorsal root ganglia may be so severe that some cells die.[39] When rat sciatic is cut and ligated in the periphery, 20–30% of the dorsal root ganglion die after a delay of 3–4 weeks. In this way a peripheral lesion is slowly converted into a partial spinal cord deafferentation by the degeneration of dorsal root afferents.

Short of frank degeneration, there are marked changes in the chemistry of the central terminals of sensory axons which have been cut rather than crushed in the periphery.[35] These centrally moving changes proceed trans-synaptically. The spinal cord cells on which the peripherally damaged afferents end lose both pre- and postsynaptic inhibitions, increase their excitability, expand their receptive fields and become spontaneously active. Central homeostatic mechanisms detect the failure of the input and raise the excitability of central cells in an attempt to compensate for the diminished input. These changes depend on transport mechanisms which are very slow by comparison with the conduction of nerve impulses. Even with the relatively short distances for transport after sciatic nerve section in the rat, the central changes do not begin for three days and reach their maximum after two weeks. Once established they are permanent. Therefore these mechanisms cannot be involved in the rapid onset phase of some neuropathic problems but they could play a part in the delayed onset pains and in the slow evolution and extension which is characteristic of both rapid and slow onset neuropathic pain.

CHANGES IN CENTRAL CONTROL MECHANISMS

Up to this point we have discussed pathological pain mechanisms as though they were a straight line of relay stations from input to output. Furthermore it has been proposed that there are control mechanisms set around each relay. Lastly it has been shown that a centrally moving wave originates from the point of damage and changes excitability successively at one station after another. This is a conceptually simple plan even though the details are quite complicated. However, the central nervous system is more than a collection of input-output lines. It certainly incorporates at a minimum, feedback systems capable not only of gain control but also of filtering and selecting the type of information flowing over the input-output lines.

An example of such a system highly relevant to neuropathic pain is mainly due to the work of McMahon.[40] The fine A delta and C afferents particularly concerned with injury detection terminate selectively on cells in the marginal layer, lamina I of the dorsal horn. These cells project mainly in the controlateral dorsolateral white matter of the spinal cord to terminate in the caudal midbrain with other targets in medulla and thalamus. The midbrain area is the indirect origin of powerful descending systems which return to the dorsal horn by way of the ipsilateral dorsolateral white matter. The effect in the cord is to facilitate the lamina I system, a positive feedback, and to inhibit the deep cells, negative feedback.

On any simple theory, this cord-brainstem-cord system would be expected to affect pain. Therefore it has been extensively investigated by many groups who have completely failed to show any effect on responses to acute noxious mechanical, thermal or chemical stimuli. A possible solution to this paradox is contained in the discovery that the rat behavioural response to peripheral nerve lesions, autotomy, is grossly exaggerated by lesions placed along the ascending or descending loops of this circuit.[41] Here we see not the expected analgesia but an increased response. In addition further work has shown that the expected decrease is indeed produced by ventral lateral white matter lesions in contrast to the dorsolateral lesions which increase the response.[42]

The existence of such long range dynamic loops may have considerable relevance to neuropathic pain in two ways. Their overall activity is likely to be set not only by the input but by the attentional set of the CNS as a whole. They are more than simple automatic volume amplification limiting feedback controls. Therefore on occasions, they could permit penetrance of pathological inputs and on other occasions they could forbid it. They are consequently a possible source of the observed variance in which the CNS has options for its reaction to inputs and may on occasions be caught unaware of a catastrophic event. The second relevance is that such circuits are famously capable of instability, the topic of Wiener's 'Cybernetics'. They have a limited normal operating range restricted by their power and temporal response characteristics. When pushed outside this range, they oscillate or flip to a fixed extreme from which they cannot restore normality. They therefore provide a possible mechanism for the observed storms of episodic pain which are such a puzzling feature of some neuropathic pains. This likelihood is increased for the lamina I-brainstem-cord loop by the finding that the circuit has a long time constant being unable to respond to acute brief inputs.

REFERENCES

1 Campbell JN, Raja SN, Cohen RH, Manning DC, Khan AA, Mayer RA. Peripheral neural mechanism of nociception. In: Melzack R, Wall PD, eds. Textbook of Pain, 2nd edn. Edinburgh: Churchill Livingstone, 1989
2 Carlen PL, Wall PD, Nadvorna MD, Steinbach T. Phantom limbs and related phenomena in recent traumatic amputations. Neurology 1978; 28: 211–217
3 Noordenbos W. Pain. Amsterdam: Elsevier, 1959
4 Tasker RR, Dostrovsky JO. Deafferentation and central pain. In: Melzack R, Wall PD, eds. Textbook of Pain, 2nd edn. Edinburgh: Churchill Livingstone, 1989
5 Sweet W. Animal models of chronic pain. Pain 1981; 10: 275–295
6 Pleasure DE. Tangier Disease. In: Dyck PJ et al. eds. Peripheral Neuropathy, Philadelphia: Saunders, 1975

7 Dyck PJ, Thomas PK, Lambert EH, eds. Peripheral Neuropathy. Philadelphia: Saunders, 1974
8 Thomas PK, Hollinrake K, Lascelles RG. The polyneuropathy of chronic renal failure. Brain 1971; 94: 761–780
9 Scadding JW. Peripheral neuropathies. In: Melzack R, Wall PD, eds. Textbook of Pain, 2nd edn. Edinburgh: Churchill Livingstone, 1989
10 Marbach JJ. Phantom tooth pain. J Endodontics 1978; 4: 362–370
11 Sharav Y. Orofacial pain. In: Melzack R, Wall PD, eds. Textbook of Pain, 2nd edn. Edinburgh: Churchill Livingstone, 1989
12 Loeser J. Atypical facial pain. In: Bonica JJ, ed. The Management of Pain, 2nd edn. Philadelphia: Lea & Febiger, 1990
13 Weddington WN, Blazer D. Atypical facial pain and trigeminal neuralgia. Psychosomatics 1979; 20: 348–359
14 Jensen TS, Rasmussen P. Pain after amputation. In: Melzack R, Wall PD, eds. Textbook of Pain, 2nd edn. Churchill Livingstone, Edinburgh, 1989
15 Sherman RA, Sherman CJ. A comparison of phantom sensations among amputees. Pain 1985; 21: 91–97
16 Bach S, Noreng MF, Tjellden NU. Phantom limb pains in amputees. Pain 1988; 33: 297–301
17 Devor M, Raber P. Heritability of symptoms in an experimental animal model of neuropathic pain. Pain 1990; 42: 51–68
18 Wall PD. Editorial. A genetic factor in the reaction of rats to peripheral nerve injury. Pain 1990; 42: 49–50
19 Noordenbos W, Wall PD. Implications of the failure of nerve resection and graft to cure chronic pain produced by nerve lesions. J Neurol Neurosurg Psychiatr 1981; 44: 1068–1073
20 Wall PD. Cord cells responding to touch damage and temperature of skin. J Neurophysiol 1960; 23: 197–210
21 Mendell LM, Wall PD. Responses of single dorsal cord cells to peripheral cutaneous unmyelinated fibres. Nature 1965; 206: 97–99
22 Hillman P, Wall PD. Inhibitory and excitatory factors controlling lamina 5 cells. Exp Brain Res 1969; 9: 284–306
23 Dubner R. Specialization in nociceptive pathways. Adv Pain Res Ther 1985; 9: 111–138
24 Cook AJ, Woolf CJ, Wall PD, McMahon SB. Expansion of cutaneous receptive fields of dorsal horn neurones following C-primary afferent fibre inputs. Nature 1987; 325: 151–153
25 Mendell LM. Physiological properties of unmyelinated fibre projections to the spinal cord. Exp Neurol 1966; 16: 316–332
26 Sugimoto T, Bennett GJ, Kajander KC. Transynaptic degeneration in the superficial dorsal horn. Pain 1990; 42: 205–214
27 Bennett GJ, Xie YK. A peripheral mononeuropathy in rat. Pain 1988; 33: 87–108
28 Wall PD, Devor M. The effect on peripheral nerve injury on dorsal root potentials and on transmission of afferent signals into the spinal cord. Brain Res 1981; 209: 95–111
29 Woolf CJ, Wall PD. Chronic peripheral nerve section diminishes the primary afferent A-fibre mediated inhibition of rat dorsal horn neurones. Brain Res 1982; 242: 77–85
30 Bromage PR, Melzack R. Phantom limbs and the body scheme. Canad Anaesth Soc J 1974; 21: 267–274
31 Cousins MJ, Bridenbaugh PO. Neural Blockade, 2nd edn. Philadelphia: Lippincott, 1988
32 Lindblom U, Meyerson BA. Influence on touch, vibration and cutaneous pain of dorsal column stimulation. Pain 1975; 1: 257–270

33 Wall PD, Sweet WH. Temporary abolition of pain in man. Science 1967; 155: 108–109
34 Devor M. The pathophysiology ofg damaged peripheral nerve. In: Melzack R, Wall PD, eds. Textbook of Pain, 2nd edn. Edinburgh: Churchill Livingstone, 1989
35 Fitzgerald M. The course and termination of primary afferent fibres. In: Melzack R, Wall PD, eds. Textbook of Pain, 2nd edn. Edinburgh: Churchill Livingstone, 1989
36 Wall PD, Mills R, Fitzgerald M, Gibson SJ. Chronic blockade of sciatic nerve transmission by tetrodotoxin does not produce central changes in the dorsal horn of the spinal cord of the rat. Neurosci Lett 1982; 30: 315–320
37 Fitzgerald M, Wall PD, Goedert M, Emson PC. Nerve growth factor counteracts the neurophysiological and neurochemical effects of chronic sciatic nerve injury. Brain Res 1985; 332: 131–141
38 Devor M, Wall PD. Plasticity in the spinal cord sensory map following peripheral nerve injury in rats. J Neurosci 1981; 1 (No. 7): 679–684
39 Ygge J. Intercostal nerve transection and its effect on the dorsal root ganglion. J Comp Neurol 1989; 279: 199–211
40 McMahon SB, Wall PD. The significance of plastic changes in lamina I systems. In: Cervero F, Bennett GJ, Headley PM, eds. Processing of Sensory Information in the Superficial Dorsal Horn of the Spinal Cord. New York: Plenum Press, 1989: pp. 249–272
41 Wall PD, Bery J, Saade NE. Effects of lesions to rat spinal cord lamina I cell projection pathways on reactions to acute and chronic noxious stimuli. Pain 1988; 35: 327–339
42 Saade NE, Atweh SF, Jabbur SJ, Wall PD. Effects of lesions in anterolateral columns and dorsolateral funiculi on autotomy and reactions to acute noxious stimuli in rats. Pain 1990; 42: 313–321

British Medical Bulletin (1991) Vol. 47, No. 3, pp. 644–666
© The British Council 1991

Neurogenic pain syndromes and their management

D Bowsher
Pain Research Institute, University Department of Neurological Science, Walton Hospital, Liverpool, UK

Neurogenic pain is defined as pain due to dysfunction of the peripheral or central nervous system, in the absence of nociceptor (nerve terminal) stimulation by trauma or disease. Other terms used to describe some (but not all) forms of neurogenic pain include neuropathic pain, deafferentation pain, and central pain; all these terms are subsumed into the wider expression 'neurogenic pain'. The clinical syndromes representing this type of disorder make up at least 25% of the patients attending most pain clinics. This is undoubtedly proportionately greater than its incidence in chronic pain as a whole, and is a measure of its intractability and of the therapeutic dilemma which it presents. However, neurogenic pain syndromes are much commoner than is perhaps generally recognized: when all categories are taken into account, there are probably more than 550,000 cases in the UK population of 56 million at any one time, i.e. a prevalence of about 1%.

Neurogenic pain, unlike nocigenic, somatogenic, or tissue-damage pain, does not arise as the result of nerve terminal excitation in damaged tissue, but because of malfunction in the peripheral or central nervous system. This may be due to physical (trauma, infection, stroke) or functional (trigeminal neuralgia, diabetic neuropathy) damage to axons. We are thus talking about painful conditions such as post-herpetic and trigeminal neuralgia, painful diabetic neuropathy, reflex sympathetic dystrophy and causalgia, and so-called 'thalamic syndrome', better called central post-stroke pain because most lesions are not in the thalamus, to name but a few; less common causes include multiple sclerosis and tabes dorsalis. Taken together, neurogenic pains are common; they account for more than 25% of all patients seen at the very large Regional (> 3000 patients p.a.) Pain-Relieving Clinic at Walton Hospital in Liverpool and of the 13 District Pain Clinics in Mersey Region and North Wales. The incidence of neurogenic pain increases with age, so that at the Regional Centre for Pain Relief in Liverpool it accounts for one third of all pain clinic patients over the age of 65, and one half of those over 70. In an ageing population, therefore, neurogenic pain must be taken very seriously.

Although the causes of neurogenic pain are legion, its manifestations and its treatment are fairly uniform. Thus despite the woefully inadequate state of knowledge about its pathophysiology, it does seem to be more or less an entity, albeit with a number of recognisable subcategories. Its main distinguishing features,[1-3] in addition to the absence of factors obviously stimulating nociceptors, are:

1. Patients frequently complain of a scalding or burning and/or less often (except in the case of trigeminal neuralgia) stabbing or shooting pain, often in addition to more familiar descriptions such as aching or throbbing. More articulate patients describe the burning as being like the paradoxical heat pain felt on plunging an extremity into very cold water or holding a snowball (ice-burn); if it can be established that the 'burning' is of this type, it is virtually pathognomonic. However, it must be emphasized that many patients with neurogenic pain do not use these shibboleth words to describe their pain. Nevertheless, pain descriptors used by patients with nocigenic (e.g. low back pain) and neurogenic (e.g. postherpetic neuralgia) pain are very different.[4,5]

2. NEUROGENIC PAIN DOES NOT RESPOND TO NARCOTIC ANALGESICS. While large doses of analgesics may 'take the edge off the pain' in a few cases, there is no real analgesic effect[1,6] short of a lowering of conscious level. While the failure of narcotics to relieve the pain is highly characteristic of neurogenic pain, it is hardly to be recommended as a method of diagnosis! It is better not to use them, having come to the correct conclusion by other means. Pain-relieving clinics have to detoxify far too many agonized geriatric junkies before rational treatment of neurogenic pain can be initiated.

3. With the exception of those neurogenic pains characterized

entirely by allodynia and shooting pains, i.e. mainly trigeminal neuralgia (and the very rare glossopharyngeal neuralgia), neurogenic pain is accompanied by a clinically evident partial sensory deficit.[3] (In fact, even in trigeminal neuralgia, subclinical sensory deficit can be detected by careful instrumental testing[7]) Thus cotton wool, thermal, and pinprick sensations may be diminished or absent in the affected area. The most frequently affected of these is thermal sensation. With an affected extremity, the patient is frequently unable to tell how hot or cold the water is in a bath or handbasin. It should be noted that the sensory deficit is usually of greater extent on the body surface than the pain; and that the painful area does not necessarily correspond to the area of maximal sensory deficit—indeed, it is quite rare for it to do so.

4. There is frequently an autonomic instability, most typically seen perhaps in the 'trophic' skin changes of causalgia, when the skin is red, shiny, and hot. Sweating is frequently affected, in either direction, so that the affected area of skin is either dryer or wetter than the corresponding area on the other side. Skin temperature too is frequently altered; contact thermography suggests that it is usually cooler (= cutaneous vasoconstriction) than the contralateral unaffected area. It is however warmer (= vasodilation) in causalgia/reflex sympathetic dystrophy, diabetic neuropathy and some cases of postherpetic neuralgia. Cutaneous vasoconstriction is the only objective autonomic change apparently found in trigeminal neuralgia (see below). It disappears when the condition is relieved by radiofrequency thermocoagulation, but reappears when and if there is a relapse into further pain.[8] This observation leads us to believe that the autonomic disturbance is intimately associated with the pain.

But the feature which most frequently emerges on questioning, or sometimes even spontaneously, is that the pain is aggravated by emotional events such as being angry or upset, and also by orgasm, as well as by a cold (or occasionally a warm) environment. By the same token, it is sometimes partly alleviated by rest, relaxation, and emotional calmness.

The autonomic instability is also shown by the fact that the patient is usually able to fall asleep as easily (or with as little difficulty) as usual, despite the severity of neurogenic pain. This is because relaxation lowers autonomic tone and so reduces pain. The lack of change in falling asleep can sometimes be difficult to elicit, because these usually elderly patients often say that they have difficulty in getting off to sleep, or can't do so without a hypnotic. However, careful questioning will usually show that this was also the case before the onset of the painful condition. These patients usually have no more difficulty in getting off to sleep than before the onset of the neurogenic pain, though they may wake in agony, perhaps during REM sleep.

5. Allodynia—the elicitation of pain by a normally non-painful stimulus—is a common feature of neurogenic pain. A good example is the trigger points of trigeminal neuralgia, when a stimulus such as the presence of food in the mouth or of the wind on the cheek may set off the pain. In a number of other conditions, rubbing may be the most effective stimulus: it is not uncommon to see post-herpetic patients who go to the most elaborate lengths to prevent their clothes from rubbing their skin. Yet firm grasping of, for example, an allodynic limb in causalgia or thalamic syndrome may not be pain-provoking, or may even relieve the pain for a moment or two. Cold allodynia is particularly common in neurogenic pains. This may be revealed by the patient's report that, 'My pain is worse when its cold'—but can easily be elicited by a cold stimulus, such as an ice cube applied to the skin. The physiology of cold allodynia has not yet been subjected to modern research.

In addition to tactile and cold allodynia, some patients exhibit movement allodynia, which occurs during isotonic or isometric muscle contraction, and may therefore arise from the activation of muscle spindle afferents. It is particularly seen in post-stroke pain, but it may also occur in those cases of trigeminal neuralgia in which the patients complain of pain elicitation by facial movement.

Tactile allodynia can be distinguished from tenderness (which is how patients often describe it) because pain is caused only by phasic light tactile stimuli, and not by firm pressure; indeed, some patients find that pain elicited by transitory stimulation is **relieved** by firm pressure. In physiological terms, allodynia is caused by stimulation of Aβ low-threshold rapidly-adapting mechanoreceptors with small receptive fields (RA II),[9] and cannot be elicited from any other type of mechanoreceptor, such as slowly-adapting (SA) receptors, activation of which may even relieve pain. Thus it may be seen, in ophthalmic post-herpetic neuralgia, when moving one hair in the eyebrow.

Allodynia occurs in 100% of cases of trigeminal neuralgia, in which it is the leading (and frequently only) complaint. Almost

90% of subjects with postherpetic neuralgia have allodynias, and it is this which usually distresses them more than anything else. More than 50% of patients with central post-stroke pain have allodynia in one form or another. Allodynia does not occur in all cases of neurogenic pain, but when it does, alone of all the characteristics listed here, it is pathognomonic.

DIAGNOSIS OF NEUROGENIC PAIN

Only two of the foregoing factors are invariably present in neurogenic pain. One is the absence of response to narcotic analgesics, but as stated above, this should never be used as a diagnostic test. The other is clinically evident sensory deficit, with the exception of those neuralgias characterized only by stabbing/shooting pain (see below); but sensory deficit can of course occur without neurogenic pain being present. A burning and/or shooting character to the pain and autonomic instability do not occur in every case either, but if they do, together with sensory deficit, there is a very strong presumption of neurogenic pain. It can be diagnosed with complete confidence if allodynia is present.

There is nothing, of course, to prevent neurogenic and nocigenic (tissue-damage) pain co-existing in the same patient. For example, malignant disease, as well as damaging tissues, may also compress peripheral nerves or the spinal cord. It is not unusual for a neurogenic pain element to be revealed as a result of the successful therapeutic elimination of tissue damage pain. Mixed pains are also seen in traumatic brachial plexus avulsion, herniated intervertebral disc, diabetes, phantom limb, and a number of other less common conditions.

NEUROGENIC PAIN SYNDROMES

These can be classified in a number of ways. It has recently become fashionable to divide neurogenic pains into sympathetic-dependent and non-sympathetic-dependent pains. This rather tautologous definition depends upon the fact that some neurogenic pains (notably causalgia/reflex sympathetic dystrophy) are relieved by sympathetic blockade. This has led some algologists to perform sympatholysis in all cases of neurogenic pain. The often disappointing results of such therapeutic attempts show that sympathetic dependence is in fact a temporal phenomenon: many neurogenic pains are relieved by sympatholysis in the early stages, but not later on. The length of time for which a neurogenic pain is 'sympathetic-dependent' varies between different neurogenic pain syndromes; causalgia, both major and minor (reflex sympathetic dystrophy), are noteworthy for remaining sympathetic-dependent for a long time. This change in response to sympatholysis betokens a dynamic change in the pathophysiology of neurogenic pain.

The simplest classification of neurogenic pain syndromes is probably anatomical, according to whether the peripheral or central nervous system is primarily affected, with an intermediate category for junctional afflictions. But wherever the seat of the primary change, the failure of destructive procedures to alleviate neurogenic pain, whether performed on peripheral nerves or spinal cord, shows that the ultimate physiopathology of neurogenic pain must reside in the central nervous system.

Peripheral neurogenic pains

There are two distinct categories of peripheral neurogenic pain. First, and somewhat apart, are those neuralgias characterized by allodynia and shooting pain alone with no sensory deficit. Secondly, there are those conditions in which the principal pain is mainly not shooting, and in which there is a sensory deficit.

Conditions characterized by shooting pain, allodynia, and no sensory deficit

Trigeminal neuralgia, in its idiopathic form, is most commonly first seen from the seventh decade onwards—but it has been observed in children, and a first attack has been reported by a subject over 100 years old. The second or third division, and very much more rarely the first, is the usual site of pain; and it is slightly commoner on the right side than the left, and in women than in men.

The first attack (like many subsequent ones) comes out of the blue. It is described as a stabbing, shooting, jabbing, lancinating, pain, 'like an electric shock' in the face, lasting only a few seconds. As the attack is so short, and the pain goes away, often not to reappear for some time, it is very rare for patients to seek medical advice after the first attack, though it should be stressed that severity (as opposed to frequency) may be maximal from the first. Further attacks occur, and their frequency increases, causing the patient to consult a doctor (or dentist). There is a 'trigger zone' from which attacks can be elicited. This is usually on the exterior of the face, but may be intra-oral. Attacks can be set off not only by touching the face, but by a puff of air, particularly cold air, when the trigger zone is external; the patient may not wash or shave the affected side of the face. In other cases, the presence of food in the mouth, or even the act of talking, may serve to trigger attacks. In the very much less common glossopharyngeal neuralgia, the spasms of pain are in the throat, frequently triggered by swallowing.

Interestingly, although the pain may radiate into the gums, it does not penetrate the teeth. This is of some theoretical importance, because trigeminal neuralgia attacks are pure allodynia. As has been stated above, allodynia occurs on stimulation of a particular category of Aβ fibres, and these are not found in teeth, though they are plentiful in the gums. Autonomic instability demonstrates itself in trigeminal neuralgia in several ways. Subjectively, the patient who while awake suffers a pain so agonising that it not infrequently leads to suicide, has no difficulty in falling asleep; and conversely suffers an increased frequency of attacks when emotionally disturbed. Objectively, there is cutaneous vasoconstriction in the affected region of the face,[10] which disappears when the pain is relieved by retrogasserian thermocoagulation.[8]

When the attacks have subsided for some time, patients may also complain of a more or less constant background ache. It has not been determined whether this is also a neurogenic pain, or a somatic pain induced in muscle by the frequent spasms.

Although idiopathic trigeminal neuralgia is a characteristic syndrome, differential diagnosis is of some importance, particularly with respect to:

1. Neuralgia due to trigeminal **nerve compression**. This can occur not only with intracerebral tumours, but with aberrant blood vessels beating against the nerve root. The symptoms are identical to idiopathic trigeminal neuralgia, but there is frequently an objectively demonstrable sensory deficit. A sign emphasized by some clinicians is exacerbation, or provocation, of the pain by leaning forward; this is thought to be caused by increase in vascular compression by the change in position. There is currently considerable debate about the pathology of trigeminal neuralgia, with some neurosurgeons arguing that there is vascular compression in the majority of cases. The

proponents of this theory advocate craniotomy and microvascular decompression in as many cases as possible.[11] However, the middle view adumbrates operation only in those otherwise healthy patients who exhibit sensory loss.

2. Symptomatic trigeminal neuralgia is a recognized complication of **multiple sclerosis**. In most cases, the patient is known to have MS long before trigeminal neuralgia develops. In cases where this diagnosis is not previously known, it may be suspected if:

(a) the patient is relatively young, and/or
(b) there is a sensory deficit in the face, and/or
(c) there is a history of visual disturbance, and/or
(d) there are changes in the optic disc on ophthalmoscopic examination, or
(e) there are any other manifestations of multiple sclerosis.

However, it should be mentioned that medical treatment is the same for trigeminal neuralgia as a complication of MS as in the idiopathic condition.

3. **Temporo-mandibular joint (TMJ) dysfunction**, which is a form of masticatory dysfunction syndrome, may mimic trigeminal neuralgia. Stabbing pains occur about 1 cm in front of the joint; they are usually associated with jaw movement, not necessarily mastication. The pains do not occur every time the jaw is moved, so may not be provoked by the examiner. However, the stabbing pain is never truly 'spontaneous' in the sense of being provoked by mechanical stimuli as slight as air-puffs. In addition to the stabbing pains, a dull ache, sometimes persisting all day, is present from the start, is characteristic of all forms of masticatory dysfunction syndrome. The patient will frequently have a mechanical jaw closure problem, perhaps associated with misaligned dentures or gingival shrinkage with age. Those given to nocturnal tooth grinding (audible) or jaw clenching (silent) are also prone to develop the condition. Geniculate herpes zoster (see below) can also cause diagnostic problems.

4. **Non-neural facial pain** ('atypical facial pain') may also be difficult to exclude on purely clinical grounds. However, contact thermography, easily and quickly performed in the clinic, fails to reveal any difference between the affected and unaffected

sides—whereas in true trigeminal neuralgia (idiopathic or symptomatic), there is almost always a cutaneous vasoconstriction.[8] If thermography is unavailable, a sensitive skin thermometer may be used, though with the small surface of the sensor, it is more difficult to be certain that there is no area of reduced skin temperature. It may be helpful to take the patient's age into consideration; the younger the patient, the more unlikely (though not impossible) is true trigeminal neuralgia.

So long as possibly serious organic disease can be ruled out, therapeutic trial with carbamazapine may be undertaken, since the drug is virtually specific for trigeminal and glossopharyngeal neuralgia. 100 mg should be taken at night for the first 3 days, then 100 mg night and morning; after the first week, the dose can be increased to 100 mg three times a day, and should be held at this level for two weeks. If the effect is insufficient, the dose can be increased by 100 mg a week up to a maximum of 800 mg. It may eventually be necessary (see below) to increase dosage up to 1200 mg/day. But at higher levels plasma concentration should be monitored; optimal levels are between 13 and a maximum of 42 μmol/l (3–10 μg/ml).

Carbamazepine is not an analgesic, so it is unusual for an effect to be seen on taking the first few doses; indeed it is not usual to see no effect for several days. It is most important to make sure the patient understands this—not only in the case of trigeminal neuralgia, but all other neurogenic pains as well (see below). Far too many patients try one or two doses of a drug and then give it up, saying, 'it didn't take the pain away, doctor', unless they are warned. They must also be warned about the possible side-effects of carbamazepine (particularly dizziness and drowsiness, less frequently gastro-intestinal disturbances; if a rash develops, they must STOP taking the drug) and assured that these are likely to pass off after the first few days. If the patient proves intolerant of carbamazepine, oxcarbamazepine may be tried, in the dose of 300 mg for every 200 mg of carbamazepine.[12]

If no effect whatsoever is obtained with full doses of carbamazepine after one month, the trial may be abandoned, and the patient sent for specialist investigation and advice, with reasonable certainty that whatever the condition is, it is not trigeminal neuralgia. More often, though, the patient may report some slight improvement after a fortnight or even a month. Provided that one can be sure that this is not being said to 'please the doctor' (and because the patient has faith in the doctor, and believes that the doctor must be making him/her better), i.e. is a placebo effect, then the dose can be gradually and cautiously increased until relief is obtained.

Although virtually self-evident, it should perhaps be stated that there is no point in carrying out a therapeutic trial until the attacks are sufficiently frequent to allow one to be certain after a couple of weeks that drugs are having an effect. By rule of thumb, this means an attack every two days or at the very least twice a week. In fact, patients do not often seek advice until this sort of frequency is attained.

The majority of cases of trigeminal neuralgia eventually escape from control by carbamazepine, even though the dose may have been increased up to about 800 mg/day or every 1200 mg/day in divided doses. Other anticonvulsants (sodium valproate [valproic acid], phenytoin) or baclofen[13] may be tried, but invasive methods are usually necessary at this stage. The method of choice is most frequently percutaneous radiofrequency differential thermocoagulation[14]; but both cryosurgey and glycerol injection[15], both effected percutaneously, are popular in some clinics. All these methods ideally spare the ophthalmic division of the nerve entirely, and also (though with less certainty) low-threshold mechanoreceptive function in the affected division(s). Hampf et al.[8] observed that following pain relief by radiofrequency thermocoagulation, the cutaneous vasoconstriction which is present in trigeminal neuralgia disappears, and remains absent up to 6 months later, provided that pain is still absent; but that if pain recurs after coagulation, so does the cutaneous vasoconstriction.

It was as long ago as 1877 that Trousseau[16] described trigeminal neuralgia as a form of 'sensory epilepsy', although anticonvulsant therapy was not used until 1942, by Bergouignan,[17] and none were really satisfactory until the advent of carbamazepine in 1962 (Blom). At the present time it may seem more practical to stand this axiom on its head and say that shooting neurogenic pains can usually be treated with anticonvulsants. This applies not only to the neuralgias currently under discussion, but also to the shooting element of the symptomatically mixed neurogenic pains described below.

Metatarsalgia (Morton's Neuralgia) is generally recognized as a true neuralgic shooting pain starting in the foot, and shooting up (and never down, like sciatica) the leg when the metatarsal region touches the ground. It is characterized by the presence of a neuroma under the matatarsal head(s), removal of which cures the condition. Like other allodynic shooting pains, it can be symptomatically treated with anticonvulsants.

Another form of shooting pain, now but rarely seen, is the *lightning pain of tabes dorsalis*. The history will usually establish the diagnosis. It is perhaps more obvious with tabes than with some other neuralgias that the pain is exacerbated (i.e. the attacks more frequent) at times of emotional stress. This is in accordance with the general rules of neurogenic pain, and serves as a reminder that neuralgias have an autonomic component. In our experience[18], the drug of first choice for tabetic crises is sodium valproate [valproic acid], in an initial dose of 200 mg at night, increasing after one week to 200 mg morning and evening, and after a further week to 200 mg three times a day after food. It is rarely necessary to go to doses higher than 600 or 800 mg/day for the control of shooting pain (in tabes dorsalis or any other condition), although for epilepsy daily doses as high as 2400 mg are used. The optimal plasma concentration is said to be from 278 to 694 μmol/l and the lower part of this range is likely to be effective for shooting pains. The drug is occasionally hepatotoxic, especially during the first few months of administration, so both clinical (vomiting, jaundice, anorexia, weakness) and serological signs of liver failure should be carefully looked for. For patients on long-term treatment with sodium valproate, many clinicians consider it prudent to carry out liver function tests every three to six months. Heartburn is a common side-effect at the beginning of treatment, about which the patient must be warned. Over the longer term, weight gain is frequent.

Three forms of curable nerve compression give rise to shooting pains. One is *prolapsed intervertebral disc (p.i.d.)* giving rise to sciatica in the lower limb. The others are *carpal* and the rare *tarsal tunnel syndromes*, affecting the upper and lower limbs respectively. If surgery has to be deferred, or for some reason cannot be performed, the exhibition of anticonvulsants can have a pain-relieving effect.

Any form of nerve compression can cause shooting pains. Thus it can occur in cancer—due to entrapment of a nerve in the tumour mass, or more frequently to compression resulting from vertebral collapse, resulting in girdle or hemigirdle pains. Vertebral collapse of course frequently occurs suddenly in cancer, giving rise to a sudden access of shooting pain for which the physician will be called. Such patients are frequently already under treatment by narcotics; but anticonvulsants should now be added. Not uncommonly, effective treatment of tissue-damage pain in malignant disease, for example by anterolateral cordotomy or by morphine delivery through an intrathecal catheter, reveals an underlying neurogenic pain.

Conditions characterized by sensory deficit and other (usually burning) pains, with or without shooting pains and allodynia

Neurogenic pains characterized by burning and perhaps shooting, together with or without other types of pain such as throbbing, aching, or squeezing (compression), or burning alone, with or without any other types of pain, form another category, to be differentiated from the pure shooting pains. There is, unfortunately, no generic name for this category of painful conditions, but they may be considered as peripheral or central neurogenic pains—it being understood that the pure shooting neuralgias are excluded. These conditions are all clinically very similar, and are mainly differentiated on the basis of history and distribution of pain.

Neurogenic pains of this type can occur in a number of systemic diseases, of which the commonest is probably painful diabetic neuropathy; vitamin B12 deficiency is another example. Generally neurogenic pain of this type should of course disappear as the underlying condition is treated; but it may prove intractable, particularly in the case of diabetic neuropathy. If it is necessary to treat these pains symptomtically, they should be treated in the same way as e.g. post-herpetic neuralgia (see below), and not with conventional analgesics.

Post-herpetic neuralgia is by far the commonest form of neurogenic pain and is said to follow one tenth of all cases of herpes zoster (itself by far the commonest disease affecting the nervous system), but more like 50% of those over 60 years of age. It usually follows directly on from shingles without a break, but there may rarely be a pain-free interval between the attack of acute zoster and the onset of painful post-herpetic neuralgia. Post-herpetic neuralgia is in fact defined as pain present one month after the rash has healed. Somewhat over half of all cases of shingles occur in thoracic dermatomes (particularly T5), another quarter in the ophthalmic division of the trigeminal nerve, up to one fifth in cervical dermatomes, and the rest elsewhere.

While the diagnosis of post-herpetic neuralgia (PHN) is usually perfectly obvious from the history, scars of the rash, distribution and description of the pain, it may occasionally present as an emergency in cases where the rash was minimal, or completely healed. There is NO relationship between the severity of acute shingles and the likelihood (or not) of developing PHN. It has, however, been suggested that there may be some correlation between the degree of sensory loss in acute shingles and the incidence of PHN.[19] There are cases of shingles in which the rash cannot be seen—the classical example is geniculate herpes, characterized by the onset of pain which is shooting in nature, and so cause confusion with trigeminal neuralgia; careful examination of the external auditory meatus (including comparison with that on the other side) will usually reveal a vesicular rash or its cicatrices.

Although the pain of PHN is typically described as burning and/or shooting, in our experience a large number of patients complain of aching, dragging, or 'boring' pains. The latter, and the absence of burning, are in our experience noteworthy in cases whose acute shingles has been treated with acyclovir. In almost 90% of cases, the painful area is exquisitely tender (allodynic) although it is in an area of partial sensory deficit[20], and patients will sometimes go to extraordinary lengths to prevent clothes moving across the affected region of skin, binding themselves into veritable cuirasses of unmovable material.

The first duty of the attending physician is to do all within his/ her power to try and stop post-herpetic neuralgia from developing. This means taking acute herpes zoster very seriously indeed; it must never be dismissed as just another irritating plague of the elderly, to be treated with sedatives, mild analgesics, and placebo. This said, it must immediately be admitted that there is no treatment of acute shingles guaranteed to prevent the development of post-herpetic neuralgia. However, antiviral treatment of acute zoster with systemic acyclovir (800 mg five times a day for 7 days) is reputed to have a good prophylactic effect on PHN[21] Immediate sympathetic blockade (where this is practicable—i.e. stellate ganglion block for ophthalmic herpes) is advocated by some. Subcutaneous infiltration of local anaesthetic, with or without steroids, is regarded as useful by many authorities. Claims have also been made for the immediate institution, as soon as the diagnosis is made, of small nocturnal doses of amitriptyline, 10 or 25 mg *nocte*, kept up for a month or two. This therapy is cheap and easy, so there would appear to be little harm in recommending that it always be tried, in addition to other measures.

The treatment of post-herpetic neuralgia is that of all neurogenic pains characterized by paradoxical burning. The most useful drugs is amitriptyline,[22] though nortriptyline and imipramine are also used. These drugs inhibit the reuptake of the neurotransmitters noradrenaline and 5-hydroxytryptamine (serotonin), and so potentiate their action. Both these transmitters are released by descending systems of supraspinal origin whose terminals are concerned with the inhibition of nociceptive circuits in the spinal cord. Since serotonin has been implicated in the activation of endogenous opioid mechanisms, and neurogenic pain is notoriously resistant to opiates, it may be that direct inhibition by noradrenergic neurones is more likely to be responsible for the therapeutic effect of amitriptyline. It may in future be found that some newer drugs in this series, facilitating only one neurotransmitter, are more effective. The ability of tricyclics to relieve neurogenic pain is independent of their antidepressant action. It is important to tell patients this, so they do not think they are being fobbed off with 'drugs for the nerves'. Like anticonvulsants, the pain-relieving effect of tricyclics is not immediate, but usually takes some weeks to develop; the patient must also be warned of this.

The commencing dose should be small—25 mg of amitriptyline (or nortriptyline) at night for younger patients, 10 mg for the elderly. Taking care not to produce side-effects, the dose should be gradually increased until the patient is taking about 75 mg a day in divided doses (50 mg for the elderly). If burning persists after a month, the dose may be cautiously increased to a maximum of 150 mg per day for younger patients—about 100 mg for the aged. Some authorities believe that phenothiazines potentiate the action of tricyclics, and so advocate the use of a proprietary preparation consisting of tablets containing 25 mg of amitriptyline and 2 mg of perphenazine; but others are opposed to this, and it is certain that the long-term effect of phenothiazines is not good, especially in the elderly.

If the aim of treatment with amitriptyline is to decrease sympathetic tone, the peripheral anticholinergic effect of the drug should be countered. Distigmine, an anticholinesterase which is said not to penetrate the blood-brain barrier, can be co-administered as two 5 mg doses daily, half an hour before meals.[23] In addition to its therapeutic effect, it has the additional bonus of decreasing the dry mouth normally produced by amitriptyline, and which is the commonest cause of non-compliance with tricyclics.

Because peripheral sympathetic overactivity seems to be implicated, and sympathetic ganglion blockade is of proven efficacy in acute shingles, sympatholysis has been much used in the treatment of PHN. In our experience, it is very disappointing in its results once the condition has become thoroughly established, i.e. more than 3 months after the appearance of the acute rash.

Many patients suffering from PHN, and other neurogenic pains in this category, also have some shooting pains, for which they should be given an anticonvulsant. Our own anticonvulsant of first choice is sodium valproate. We start with 200 mg at night and increase gradually to 200 mg two or three times a day; it is rarely necessary to go above 800 mg a day to combat the shooting pains of post-herpetic neuralgia. Combined amitriptyline-valproate therapy for PHN was first advocated for PHN by Raftery.[24] If no relief is obtained with valproate after a month, other anticonvulsants (carbamazepine, phenytoin) should be tried.

Topical therapy may be called for in many cases of post-herpetic neuralgia. Transcutaneous electrical nerve stimulation (TENS) can be surprisingly effective, provided the physician takes the trouble diligently to search for the most effective electrode sites and stimulation parameters. However, when sensory loss is such that there are insufficient large (Aβ) cutaneous fibres to stimulate, TENS will be of no benefit. As a rule of thumb, if the patient cannot feel the application of a moving pledgelet of cotton wool in the affected area, there is little point in trying TENS. It should be pointed out that TENS works, are least in part, through non-opioidergic local circuit interneurones in the spinal dorsal horn. Acupuncture, on the other hand, involves opioidergic interneurones, and therefore is not surprisingly of little value in opioid-resistant neurogenic pains such as PHN.[25]

In patients who can tolerate it, a lotion consisting of 4% dispersible aspirin in chloroform has been found effective in some cases[26]; others have benefitted form the application of benzydamine[27,28] or EMLA creams.[29] One of the commonest forms of autonomic dysfunction in PHN is anhidrosis or hypohidrosis of the affected area, which means that the affected area of skin will be very dry. In addition to the topical drugs mentioned, therefore, the patient will experience increased comfort if the skin is kept moist with substances such as oil or emollient cream (e.g. E45).

While sympathetic blockade is undoubtedly useful in acute shingles, we have been disappointed in its effects (or lack of them) on PHN. Surgical treatment by dorsal root entry zone (DREZ) microlesions are reported to have proved helpful in particularly intractable cases[30], though only for a limited time; and recently developed techniques for percutaneous differential thermocoagulation of dorsal root ganglia[31] may hopefully be expected to be useful. However, it must be remembered that although shingles begins as an infection of dorsal root ganglia and peripheral nerves by the chickenpox virus, the pathophysiology of pain in PHN must be seated deep within the central nervous system, as witnessed by the failure of destructive procedures such as dorsal (posterior) rhizotomy and even anterolateral cordotomy to relieve the pain.[32]

If the patient demands an analgesic (and they usually do), dihydrocodeine occasionally 'takes the edge off' the pain. It is the only analgesic we would be prepared to use; if its use is to be prolonged, its constipating effects must be countered, particularly in the elderly.

The importance of vigorously instituting suitable treatment at the earliest possible moment cannot be sufficiently emphasized. The longer the condition is allowed to continue, the more difficult it becomes to treat effectively; a 90% relief rate can be expected in patients treated within 3 months of the acute rash, but this drops to 30% after a year.[33] This is really why both herpes zoster and post-herpetic neuralgia (and indeed any other neurogenic pain) should be considered as neurological emergencies.

Painful diabetic neuropathy is by far the commonest of the neuropathies producing neurogenic pain. Diabetic subjects are of course prone to a number of tissue-damaged pains, such as arthropathy; but it has been estimated that about 25% of them suffer from neurogenic pain.[34] In addition to careful diabetic control, medical treatment follows the same lines as for PHN. If pain is relieved by the intravenous administration of 200 mg of lignocaine (lidocaine),[35] good results have been reported as a result of oral medication with mexiletine (400 mg, followed by 200 mg 4-hourly).[36] When this therapy is commenced, it should be performed in hospital with very frequent (or continuous) blood-pressure monitoring.

Some painful mononeuropathies resulting from pressure on

nerves are characterized more frequently by paradoxical burning rather than shooting pains. These include compression of the anterior or lateral cutaneous nerves of the thigh under the inguinal ligament (*meralgia paraesthetica*), and abdominal nerve entrapment in the rectus sheath.[37] These conditions can be relieved by amitriptyline if surgery and/or weight reduction are not feasible.

Causalgia is a classical form of peripheral neurogenic pain, usually affecting a single nerve, most frequently the median or ulnar and less often the femoral. The agonizing, typically burning, pain follows injury, always partial, to the nerve. While most cases are traumatic in origin, the impression is growing that there seems to be an increasing incidence of iatrogenic cases, consequent upon ulnar nerve transposition or lumbar disc surgery. There is almost always an interval of time between nerve injury and the onset of causalgic pain. The name causalgia minor has recently been applied to those distal forms of the condition which follow trauma such as Colles' fracture, and are more familiar under the name of reflex sympathetic dystrophy or Sudek's atrophy.

In addition to the spontaneous pain, allodynia is nearly always marked—the patient cannot bear to be touched in the affected area; there are trophic changes in the skin, including autonomic dysfunction. It has been reported that the subcutaneous injection of 1 µg of adrenaline, totally without effect in normal skin, brings on severe causalgic pain when performed in an affected area,[38] thus underlining the important role of the sympathetic nervous system in the generation of neurogenic pain. In reflex sympathetic dystrophy or causalgia minor, there is usually also osteolysis.

While the medical treatment used for postherpetic neuralgia may give some relief in causalgia, sympatholysis is the treatment of choice, unlike the case of late PHN; in other words, causalgia (major and minor), remains sympathetic-dependent (see above) for considerably longer than does PHN.

If only the distal part of a limb is affected by causalgia, depletion of adrenergic nerve terminals can be effected by the intravenous injection of guanethidine (or reserpine in those countries where guanethidine is unavailable) distal to a tourniquet; it is frequently necessary to repeat this at short intervals over two or three weeks in order to achieve a permanent result. When the upper parts of limbs are involved, it will be necessary to undertake sympatholytic injection of stellate or lumbar ganglia. Good results have been reported from medical treatment with the systemic administration of phenoxybenzamine, 10 mg t.d.s., increasing to 80 mg/day, for not more than a month[39]; but as in the case of mexilitene, the treatment has to be undertaken in hospital because of the resultant hypotension. Along the same lines, some success has been obtained in causalgia minor by treatment with ketanserin, an α1 and 5-HT2 blocker.

Transitional neurogenic pain

Intermediate between peripheral and central neurogenic pain is **brachial plexus avulsion** (or indeed any other root avulsion), most often seen after motor-cycle accidents and other trauma. While the motor deficit due to lower motor neurone damage becomes apparent immediately, the severe burning pain may not appear until a certain time has passed—often after the patient has been discharged from a traumatology service. The pain is often felt in parts of the limb entirely bereft of sensation, and so is akin to phantom limb pain following amputation. In other (more frequent) cases, the pain occurs in a part of the limb in which the sensory deficit is subtotal. Sympatholysis (stellate ganglion blockade) should if possible be carried out prophylactically in the traumatology service, since it may prevent the later onset of neurogenic pain (as in the case of acute ophthalmic shingles and PHN); and it should certainly be performed as soon as the patient complains of neurogenic pain, and repeated at frequent intervals until the patient is pain-free. Simultaneous medical treatment with amitriptyline and perhaps anticonvulsants (if shooting pains are also present) should also be instituted. As in the case of phantom limb pain, dorsal column stimulation may be of great benefit. Microlesions placed neurosurgically in the dorsal root entry zone (DREZ) of the spinal cord are said by its proponents to be helpful—and have also been used in other forms of neurogenic pain, such as post-herpetic neuralgia.

Phantom limb pain is more obviously central, and may be entirely neurogenic, in which case it should be treated in the same way as avulsion. More frequently, it is a mixture of neurogenic (as defined here) and other pain, in which the burning and shooting features may be less evident. Thus there may be a tender neuroma requiring injection or excision. Where peripheral nerve stimulation is practicable, it may be helpful. More often, it is necessary to stimulate the dorsal columns in order to reach the Aβ primary afferents ordinarily stimulated by TENS. Non-neurogenic stump pain may require treatment by conventional means.

Central neurogenic pain

Approximately one quarter of stroke subjects have a partial somatosensory deficit in addition to a motor disorder; indeed many find the somatosensory deficit more debilitating than the motor inconvenience. Between 1% and 2% of stroke victims develop spontaneous central pain. Since there are about 100,000 strokes p.a. in the U.K., this is a considerable number. Pain following a cerebral vascular accident is usualy called thalamic pain, or **thalamic syndrome**, because the first three cases described all had lesions in the thalamic somatosensory relay nucleus.[40] Since computerized axial tomography has apparently shown that in many cases the lesion is not in the thalamus[41-43], but in pathways leading to or from the somatosensory thalamus, the condition is now known as **central post-stroke pain (CPSP)**. It can follow not only classical 'stroke', but also surgically-treated subarachnoid haemorrhage,[41] tumour removal, and even head injury.

In any event, clinically the patients are victims of a cerebrovascular accident (CVA) of some sort or another. There is a tendency for their median age to be younger (about 55) than that of the 'average' stroke patient. Often also the motor effects of the stroke are not particularly severe. In about 50% of cases, the pain is felt from the time that the stroke becomes complete, or very shortly afterwards; in the other half, the pain, often burning, sometimes also shooting, but not infrequently an 'indescribable' pain brought on by movement and absent when the subject is completely still (movement allodynia), comes on any time up to 18 months after the CVA. This means that many cases of CPSP first come to the attention of the geriatrician or the family practitioner rather than to that of the neurologist.

As in pure motor stroke, the pain may involve a complete body half (or the face on one side and the trunk and limbs on the other), or just the limbs, or just the extremities of the limbs, or the whole or part of a single limb; or a small area on the face, or rarely even on the trunk. The severity of the pain varies from one case to another; it may be little worse than bad 'pins and needles', or it may be excruciating. There is always a partial sensory deficit (particularly for thermal sensation), but the pain is not necessarily coextensive with the whole area of sensory deficit, or even necessarily in the area of maximal sensory deficit. In classical 'thalamic' cases, due to infarction in the territory of the posterior cerebral artery, there is also a visual field deficit.

Allodynia occurs in about 50% of cases. Autonomic dysfunction, in terms of cutaneous vasoconstriction, sometimes of sweating anomalies in the affected area, and of exacerbation by stress and cold and alleviation by rest and sleep, can always be detected.

Treatment is as for other neurogenic pains: peripheral sympathetic blockade where feasible (and as early as possible), combined with medical treatment with amitriptyline, and anticonvulsants when shooting pain or severe 'pins and needles' are a feature. Peripheral sympathetic blockade has been of benefit in some cases.[45] In our experience, this is more effective earlier (in the sympathetic-dependent phase), but pain relief, at least for a relatively short period of time, may be seen following repeated sympathetic blockade (e.g. 48-hourly for 2 weeks). TENS has proved useful in a number of cases.[46] Large vasoconstricted areas, such as a limb, sometimes feel subjectively, as well as objectively, cold. In such cases, the vasoconstriction and feeling of coldness can be reversed by the exhibition of small doses of a peripherally-acting calcium channel blocker, such as nifedipine 10 mg t.d.s. This always increases the patient's comfort, even when it does not, of itself, relieve the pain. It was presumably because of its reputed vasodilatory effect that large doses of intravenous naloxone were recommended for the treatment of CPSP,[47] though in our experience this particular drug is of little therapeutic value.[48] Although the majority of cases of CPSP, and indeed of peripheral neurogenic pains, manifest cutaneous vasoconstriction, in a small number of cases autonomic instability is characterized by cutaneous vasodilation. In such cases, it has been suggested[49] that propranolol, a β-blocker with peripheral vasoconstrictive properties, should be used rather than vasodilator drugs such as calcium channel blockers.

As in pure motor stroke, tissue-damage pains such as that of frozen shoulder are not uncommon, in addition to neurogenic pain. They must of course be treated in the usual way, preferably by local injection of local anaesthetic and steroid, or by mobilization, physiotherapy, and non-steroidal anti-inflammatory drugs.

Central neurogenic pain has occasionally been reported in conditions other than cerebral vascular accident. The commonest are incomplete transection of the spinal cord, post-cordotomy dysaesthesia in cases of long survival, multiple sclerosis, and syringomyelia. These difficult cases should be treated in the same way as those of vascular origin.

CONCLUSIONS

1. With a little experience, it is relatively easy to recognize neurogenic pain by the simple criteria outlined here, though of course it may be more difficult in cases exhibiting mixed neurogenic and tissue-damage pains.

2. As soon as neurogenic pain is recognized, treatment with amitriptyline should be instituted. Other drugs and procedures such as sympatholysis should follow soon after. Early treatment is often effective; the longer it is delayed, the lower the proportion of cases in whom pain is relieved.

3. Never waste valuable time by initiating treatment with conventional analgesics. Once amitriptyline has been started, various forms of topical medication may be useful in peripheral neurogenic pains; and codeine may provide some alleviation by its central action.

4. The fact that none of these measures is universally successful underlines the fact that the mechanism of neurogenic pain is not yet fully understood. However, a start has been made in the recognition that clinical syndromes of apparently very diverse origin apparently have a larger similar physiopathology. Much research nevertheless remains to be done before a completely rational therapy can be undertaken.

REFERENCES

1 Bowsher D. Pain mechanisms in man. Med Times 1986; 114: 83–96
2 Bowsher D. Neurogenic Pain: Diagnosis and Treatment. Res Staff Phys 1988; 34: 23–29
3 Bowsher D. Pain Mechanisms. In: Swash M, Oxbury J eds. Textbook of Neurology. Edinburgh: Churchill Livingstone, 1991
4 Madan B, Ramamoorthy C, Bowsher D, Wells C. A survey of intractable low back pain in a pain relief clinic and some comparisons with painful osteoarthritis and postherpetic neuralgia. Schmerz Pain Douleur 1988; 9: 116–120
5 Cossins L. Features of commonest diagnoses in 1017 successive pain clinic cases. Pain 1990; (suppl 5): S350
6 Arner S, Meyerson BA. Lack of analgesic effect of opioids on neuropathic and idiopathic forms of pain. Pain 1988; 33: 11–23
7 Nurmikko T. Altered cutaneous sensation in trigeminal ralgia. Arch Neurol 1991 (in press)
8 Hampf G, Bowsler D, Wells C, Miles J. Sensory and autonomic measurements

in idiopathic trigeminal neuralgia before and after radiofrequency coagulation: Differentiation from some other causes of facial pain. Pain 1990; 40: 241–248

9 Nurmikko T, Wells C, Bowsher D. Pain and allodynia in postherpetic neuralgia: Role of somatic and sympathetic nervous systems. Acta Neurol Scand 1991 (in press)

10 Hardy PAJ, Bowsher D. Contact thermography in idiopathic trigeminal neuralgia and other facial pains. Br J Neurosurg 1989; 3: 399–402

11 Janetta PJ. Arterial compression of the trigeminal nerve at the pons in patients with trigeminal neuralgia. J Neurosurg 1967; 26: 159–162

12 Zakrzewska JM, Patsalos PN. Oxcarbazepine: A new drug in the management of intractable trigeminal neuralgia. J Neurol Neurosurg Psychiatr 1989; 52: 472–476

13 Fromm GH. The Medical and Surgical Management of Trigeminal Neuralgia. New York: Futura, 1987

14 Sweet WH, Wepsic JG. Controlled thermocoagulation of trigeminal ganglion and rootlets for differential destruction of pain fibers. J Neurosurg 1974; 40: 143–156

15 Håkansson S. Trigeminal neuralgia treated by injection of glycerol into the trigeminal cistern. Neurosurgery 1981; 9: 638–646

16 Trousseau A. Clinique médicale de l'Hôtel-Dieu de Paris. Paris: Baillière et Fils, 1877

17 Bergouignan M. Cures heureuses de névralgies faciales essentielles par le diphenyl-hydantoinate de soude. Rev Laryngol Otol Rhinol 1942; 63: 34–41

18 Bowsher D, Rennie I, Lahuerta J, Nelson A. A case of Tabes Dorsalis with tonic pupils and lightning pains relieved by sodium valproate. J Neurol Neurosurg Psychiatr 1987; 50: 239–241

19 Nurmikko T. Clinical and neurophysiological observations on acute herpes zoster. Clin J Pain 1990; 6: 284–290

20 Nurmikko T, Bowsher D. Somatosensory findings in postherpetic neuralgia. J Neurol Neurosurg Psychiatr 1990; 53: 135–141

21 Crooks RJ, Bell AR, Fiddian AP. Treatment of shingles and post-herpetic neuralgia. Br Med J 1989; 299: 392–393

22 Watson CP, Evans RJ, Reed K, Merskey H, Goldsmith L, Warsh J. Amitriptyline versus placebo in postherpetic neuralgia. Neurology 1982; 32: 671–673

23 Hampf G, Bowsher D, Nurmikko T. Amitryptiline and anticholinesterases in the treatment of chronic pain. Anaesth Progr 1989; 36: 58–62

24 Raftery H. The management of post herpetic pain using sodium valproate and amitriptyline. J Irish Med Assoc 1979; 72: 399–401

25 Lewith GT, Field J, Machin D. Acupuncture compared with placebo in post-herpetic neuralgia Pain 1983; 17: 361–368

26 King RB. Concerning the management of pain associated with herpes zoster and of postherpetic neuralgia. Pain 1988; 33: 73–78

27 Alexander JI. The use of benzydamine cream in post-herpetic neuralgia. Res Clin Forums 1988; 10: 59–64

28 Coniam SW, Hunton J. A study of benzydamine cream in post-herpetic neuralgia. Res Clin Forums 1988; 10: 65–68

29 Stow PJ, Glynn CJ, Minor B. EMLA cream in the treatment of postherpetic neuralgia. Efficacy and pharmacokinetic profile. Pain 1989; 39: 301–306

30 Friedman AH, Nashold BS, Ovelmen-Levitt J. Dorsal root entry zone lesions for the treatment of post herpetic neuralgia. J Neurosurg 1984; 60: 1258–1262

31 Nash TP. Percutaneous radiofrequency lesioning of dorsal root ganglia for intractable pain. Pain 1986; 24: 67–74

32 White JC, Sweet WH. Pain and the Neurosurgeon. Springfield, Ill: Charles C. Thomas, 1969

33 Bhala BB, Ramamoorthy C, Bowsher D, Yelnoorker KN. Shingles and post-herpetic neuralgia. Clin J Pain 1988; 4: 169–174

34 Chan AW, MacFarlane IA, Griffiths K, Wells JCD, Bowsher D. Unrecognised and untreated chronic pain in the diabetic clinic. Diabetic Med 1988; 5: 22A

35 Boas RA, Covino BG, Shanharian A. Analgesic response to i.v. lignocaine. Br J Anaesth 1982; 54: 501–505

36 Dejgard A, Petersen P, Kastrup J. Mexiletine for treatment of chronic painful diabetic neuropathy. Lancet 1988; 1: 9–11

37 Applegate WV. Abdominal cutaneous nerve entrapment syndrome. Surgery 1972; 71: 118–124

38 Torebjörk HF, Hallin RG. Microneurographic studies of peripheral pain mechanisms in man. Adv Pain Res Ther 1979; 3: 121–131

39 Ghostine SY, Comair YG, Turner DM, Kassell NF, Azar CG. Phenoxybenzamine in the treatment of causalgia. J Neurosurg 1984; 60: 1263–1268

40 Dejerine J, Roussy J. Le syndrome thalamique. Rev Neurol 1906; 14: 521–532

41 Agnew DC, Shetter AG, Segall HD, Flom RA. Thalamic pain. Adv Pain Res Ther 1983; 5: 941–946

42 Bowsher D, Lahuerta J. Central pain in 22 patients: Clinical features, somatosensory changes, and CT-scan findings. J Neurol 1985; 232 (Suppl): 297

43 Bowsher D, Lahuerta J, Brock LG. Twelve cases of central pain, only three with thalamic lesions. Pain 1984; (Suppl 2): 83

44 Bowsher D, Foy P, Shaw MDM. Central pain following subarachnoid haemorrhage and surgery. Br J Neurosurg 1989; 3: 445–452

45 Loh L, Nathan PW, Schott GD. Pain due to lesions of the central nervous system removed by sympathetic block. Br Med J 1981; 282: 1026–1028

46 Leijon G, Boivie J. Central post-stroke pain—the effect of high and low frequency TENS. Pain 1989; 88: 187–192

47 Budd K. The use of the opiate antagonist naloxone in the treatment of intractable pain. Neuropeptides 1985; 5: 419–422

48 Bainton T, Fox M, Bowsher D, Wells C. A double-blind trial of naloxone in central post-stroke pain. Possible role of blood flow. (Submitted for publication)

49 Tourian AY. Narcotic responsive 'thalamic' pain: treatment with propranolol and tricyclic antidepressants. Pain 1987; (Suppl 4): S411

British Medical Bulletin (1991) Vol. 47, No. 3, pp. 667–675
© The British Council 1991

Development of pain mechanisms

M Fitzgerald
Department of Anatomy & Developmental Biology, University College London, London, UK

Interest in the neural development of pain pathways and of the perception and treatment of pain in newborn infants has increased markedly in the last few years. The tremendous improvement in the survival of premature infants, particularly those weighing less than 1000 gm at birth, means that there are now a significant number of infants, many of whom require surgery, undergoing necessarily extensive traumatic procedures in intensive care units. At the same time it is becoming clear that the traditional belief of paediatricians and anaesthetists that newborn infants do not feel or remember pain and therefore need no anaesthesia or analgesia is rooted in a mixture of misconception and fear.[1]

The fear is a practical one arising from potential intraoperative hypotension caused by anaesthesia of infants, postanaesthesia apnea and the respiratory depression that might result from narcotic analgesia. A great number of studies have now been undertaken on the use of inhalation and intravenous anaesthetics as well as sedatives and narcotics.[2,3] Furthermore the use of spinal anaesthesia in newborn infants is now well established.[4,5] There is now sufficient information to permit rational management of paediatric pain.

The misconceptions may have arisen from early reports that babies do not feel pain based on poorly designed trials with no controls, and no definition of either the stimuli or the responses measured.[6,7] There are now a considerable number of carefully executed studies demonstrating that even the smallest preterm infant is capable of displaying pain responses (for reviews *see* References [8–11]). One recent example shows neonatal facial activity to be a good indicator of acute pain responsiveness to intramuscular injection.[12] Another demonstrates, using the flexion reflex threshold as a measure of cutaneous sensitivity,[13] a hyperalgesia that lasts for days and weeks in premature and term infants following repeated heel lances.[14] A sensitization of the heart rate response to repeated noxious stimuli has also recently been demonstrated.[15]

The extent to which the pain is understood and remembered in the newborn remains an area for psychologists but what the above studies show is that the important questions are no longer to do with whether or not babies feel pain. They clearly respond to painful stimuli and what we need to concentrate on now is: (a) how to measure those responses; and (b) what neurobiological mechanisms underlie them.

The aim of this chapter is to discuss the latter question. Until we really understand how the somatosensory system and the pathways and processes involved in pain transmission develop in the fetus and neonate we cannot expect to be able to understand and control pain in infants.

Defining the problems

Much of our knowledge of the developing mammalian nervous system comes from the laboratory rat but comparison of rat and human developmental timetables[16] suggests that the first postnatal weeks in the rat corresponds to 24 weeks gestation to the early neonatal period in humans.

By the time a rat is born many of the basic sensory and motor connections at the segmental level have already formed. Peripheral innervation is well-established, if not mature, and dorsal roots have grown into the spinal cord and formed simple reflex connections with motorneurones. For further details of these early events, *see* References [16-19] To consider the development of pain mechanisms, we need to concentrate on later phases in the development and organization of the somatosensory system. These include the maturation of primary sensory neurons, their terminals and synaptic connections in the spinal cord, the development of central circuits and transmitter-receptor interactions, the growth of long ascending projections and connections in brainstem, thalamus and cortex and the development of descending controls from higher centres back down to the spinal cord. Last but not least, we need to consider whether the normal development of these events is affected by the presence of abnormal or excessive sensory stimuli as might occur in prematurity or through invasive clinical procedures.

Maturation of peripheral primary sensory terminals

While the innervation of the skin begins in fetal life[19] it takes a long time to mature. Initially the cutaneous plexus penetrates to the surface of the epidermis but as the skin matures this plexus becomes subepidermal.[19,20] From the earliest stage of innervation, even before the development of specialized end organs, it is possible to record primary afferents responding to skin stimulation with discrete receptive fields and well-defined firing patterns.[21] Responses of low threshold afferents are amplified and given dynamic sensitivity by the innervation of specific end organs, such as hair follicles, but this does not begin until 22 weeks in the human fetus and at P7 in the rat hindlimb.[22] Polymodal nociceptors, responding to noxious mechanical, thermal and chemical stimuli are also observed as soon as the skin is innervated but unlike the low threshold responses are mature in their firing characteristics from that time.[21,24]

Despite early maturation of their afferent receptor properties, the efferent function of C fibres in producing neurogenic extravasation, via an axon reflex mechanism, does not develop in rat skin until the second postnatal week.[25]

Expression of chemical markers and putative neurotransmitters in primary sensory neurons occurs about the time or shortly after target innervation in the rat,[26] although somewhat later in the human at between 12 and 16 weeks.[26-28] Levels are low initially and gradually increase over the late fetal and postnatal period in both species.

Maturation of central primary afferent terminals and synaptic connections

In the rat spinal cord, large diameter, low threshold afferents grow into the spinal cord in advance of C fibre afferents.[29] C fibre synaptic boutons are not observed in the cord until postnatally[30] and, unlike A fibres which form synaptic connections in the spinal cord soon after growing into the grey matter,[31] take a week before they produce spikes in postsynaptic dorsal horn cells.[16,32] Before that time they are capable of producing long-lasting, subthreshold depolarizations in the cord[33] and sensitization to subsequent stimuli[16] but not the rapid bursts of spikes that are normally evoked by C fibres in the adult cord. Whether C fibre afferent terminals mature equally slowly in the human spinal cord is not known. However, it is interesting to note that there are two phases of intense synaptic development in developing human cord, one at 9–10 weeks (the period of initial reflex connections) and the other at 17–21 weeks.[34]

Development of local circuits

The anatomical development of the rat spinal cord and dorsal horn at the segmental level has been well described and the basic cellular organization is established at birth although there is considerable postnatal axonal and dendritic growth and synaptogenesis.[17] Of particular importance is that the interneurones of substantia gelatinosa do not begin their axonal and dendritic development until the postnatal period and it is not complete until P20.[35] The maturation of this area has not been studied in detail in man but by 30 weeks the main features of the adult cord are present.[36]

Physiological studies of dorsal horn cells in the neonatal period shows that while synaptic connections with primary sensory neurons are still weak, single peripheral stimuli can cause long-lasting excitation lasting minutes.[37] Furthermore the cutaneous receptive fields of dorsal horn cells are large in the newborn and gradually diminish over the first 2 postnatal weeks.[37] These properties are consistent with the well-described exaggerated cutaneous reflexes observed in the newborn rat and human infant.[13,38]

There is also considerable postnatal development of transmitter receptor systems in the dorsal horn. Enkephalin which is contained in some of these interneurons does not appear in the dorsal horn of the spinal cord until birth and then at very low levels.[24] Levels do not reach that of the adult until P15. In the human spinal cord it is one of the last peptides to appear at 12–14 weeks.[39] Opiate receptors also undergo postnatal changes in rat cord. Kappa-receptors develop first followed by the appearance of high-affinity μ-receptor binding, coinciding with the onset of κ- and μ-mediated analgesia.[40,41]

Substance P receptors are diffusely distributed in high density all over the spinal grey matter until P15 in the rat and only then become progressively more concentrated in the superficial dorsal horn and other regions.[42]

Development of descending inhibition

Descending axons from brainstem projection neurons appear to grow down the spinal cord early in fetal life.[43] These axons may not, however, extend collaterals into the dorsal horn to influence sensory processing for some considerable time.[44] Furthermore, the development of appropriate neurotransmitters in descending pathways such as 5-HT (serotonin) and noradrenaline is an important consideration. In the rat the first serotonergic axons are observed in the white matter at E18 and have entered the grey matter at birth, although are still very sparse and diffuse at this stage.[45] An adult pattern of serotonergic innervation in the cord is not achieved until P14 in the cervical cord and P21 in the lumbar cord. Noradrenaline containing terminals appear earlier in the dorsal horn than serotonin at about P4[46,47] and levels are mature by approximately 2 postnatal weeks. Again, it is found in the ventral horn well before this.

Electrophysiological recording from rat dorsal horn neurons of the inhibition of afferent-evoked activity by electrical stimulation of descending fibres in the dorsolateral funiculus (DLF),[48] shows no descending inhibition until P10. Only by P19 did the inhibition from DLF stimulation resemble that seen in the adult.

Development of pain mechanisms in higher centres

Little is known of the maturation of projection pathways, thalamic and cortical connections in relation to pain processing. In the rat, evoked potentials in the somatosensory cortex from the forepaw develop the adult form by P12.[49] Evoked potentials in humans suggest that thalamic inputs reach the cortex at 29 weeks[50] and this is supported by anatomical studies.[51] Unfortunately such evidence of sensory inputs to the cortex tells us little about the integration or analysis of noxious information at this time.

Central consequences of peripheral injury

In the clinical context, acute infant pain will be associated with invasive or traumatic procedures. The developing nervous system is extremely vulnerable to peripheral injury. Section of a single nerve in the new born rat has considerable, irreversible sensory consequences. The majority of the dorsal root ganglion cells die,[52] and as a result the central dorsal root terminals of nearby intact nerves sprout in the spinal cord to occupy areas normally exclusively devoted to the deafferented nerve.[53] These new sprouts form functional connections with inappropriate dorsal horn cells in areas way outside their normal termination area.[54] As a result the nervous system becomes permanently distorted with a far greater than normal amount devoted to inputs surrounding the denervated skin. This may be a useful adaptive response acting to compensate for lost sensory input from a region of the body surface but we cannot be sure that the long term consequences on sensory perception are beneficial. Certainly the effects of nerve injury early in rat development are not restricted to the primary afferents but spread to postsynaptic dorsal horn cells[55] up through higher levels of the nervous system, e.g. cortex[56,57] and pyramidal tract,[58] suggesting that invasive procedures affecting the nervous system of the premature infant should be undertaken only with extreme caution.

CONCLUSIONS

Although basic somatosensory pathways are formed by birth there is considerable postnatal development in relation to pain pathways. In particular C afferents are unable to produce rapid reactions in postsynaptic cells, only slow long-lasting sensitizing effects. As a result, nociceptive inputs may produce responses in the CNS but these may not always be sufficiently organized to produce predictable behavioural reactions. Furthermore the lack of descending and segmental inhibition in the neonatal cord implies that there is less endogenous control of noxious inputs. As a result noxious inputs may have an even more profound effect than in the adult but the reactions will be more diffuse and the effects potentially underestimated. This, together with the vulnerability of the developing nervous system to local peripheral damage means that pain and injury in the newborn must be taken seriously.

REFERENCES

1 Purcell-Jones G, Dormon F, Sumner E. Paediatric anaesthetists' perceptions of neonatal and infant pain. Pain 1988; 33: 181–188
2 Berde CB. The treatment of pain in children. Pain 1990; (Suppl 5): S3
3 Anand KJS, Sippell WG, Aynsley-Green A. Randomized trial of fentanyl anaesthesia in preterm babies undergoing surgery: effects on the stress response. Lancet 1987; 62–66
4 Berry FA, Gregory GA. Do premature infants require anesthesia for surgery? Anesthesiology 1987; 67: 291–293
5 Welborn LG, Rice LJ, Hannallah RS, Broadman LM, Ruttimann UE, Fink

R. Postoperative apnea in former preterm infants: prospective comparison of spinal and general anaesthesia. Anesthesiology 1990; 12: 838–842

6 McGaw MB. Neural maturation as exemplified in the changing reactions of the infant to pinprick. Child Dev 1941; 12: 31–42

7 Merskey H. On the development of pain. Headache 1970; 10: 116–123

8 Owens ME. Pain in infancy: conceptual and methodological issues. Pain 1984; 20: 213–230

9 McGrath PJ, Unruh AM. Pain in children and adolescents. Pain research and clinical management, vol. 1. Amsterdam: Elsevier, 1987: pp. 47–128

10 Anand KJS, Hickey PR. Pain and its effects in the human neonate and fetus N Engl J Med 317: 1321–1329

11 Fitzgerald M. Pain and analgesia in neonates. Trends Neurosci 1987; 9: 254–256

12 Grunau RVE, Johnston CC, Craig KD. Neonatal facial and cry responses to invasive and non-invasive procedures. Pain 1990; 42: 295–306

13 Fitzgerald M, Shaw A, MacIntosh N. Postnatal development of the cutaneous flexor reflex: comparative study of preterm infants and newborn rat pups. Dev Med Child Neurol 1988; 30: 520–526

14 Fitzgerald M, Millard C, McIntosh N. Cutaneous hypersensitivity following peripheral tissue damage in newborn infants and its reversal with topical anaesthesia. Pain 1989; 39: 31–36

15 Booth JC, McGrath PA, Brigham MC, Frewen T, Whittall S. Critically ill neonates distress responses during invasive medical procedures. Pain 1990; (Suppl. 5): S28

16 Fitzgerald M. The developmental neurobiology of pain. In: Bond M, Woolf CJ, Charlton M, eds. Proceedings VIth World Congress on Pain. 1990: (In press)

17 Altman J, Bayer SA. The development of the rat spinal cord. Adv Anat Embryol Cell Biol 1984; 85: 1–166

18 Fitzgerald M, Reynolds ML, Benowitz LI. GAP-43 expression in the developing rat lumbar cord. Neurosci. 1991; 41: 187–199

19 Reynolds ML, Fitzgerald M, Benowitz LI. GAP-43 expression in the developing hindlimb. Neuroscience 1991; 41: 201–211

20 Fitzgerald MJT. Perinatal changes in epidermal innervation in rat and mouse. J Comp Neurol 1966; 126: 37–42

21 Fitzgerald M. Spontaneous and evoked activity of fetal primary afferents 'in vivo'. Nature 1987; 326: 603–605

22 Payne J, Middleton J, Fitzgerald M. The morphological development of sensory innervation of hairs in the rat pup and human infant. (Submitted)

23 Nurse CA, Diamond J. A fluorescent microscopic study of the development of rat touch domes and their Merkel cells. Neuroscience 1984; 11: 509–520

24 Fitzgerald M. Cutaneous primary afferent properties in the hindlimb of the neonatal rat. J Physiol 1987; 383: 79–92

25 Fitzgerald M, Gibson S. The physiological and neurochemical development of peripheral sensory C fibres. Neuroscience 1984; 13: 933–344

26 Marti E, Gibson SJ, Polak JM, et al. Ontogeny of peptide- and amine-containing neurones in motor, sensory and autonomic regions of rat and human spinal cord, dorsal root ganglia and rat skin. J Comp Neurol 1987; 266: 332–359

27 Charnay Y, Chayvialle JA, Pradayrol L, Bouvier R, Paulin C, Dubois PM. Ontogeny of somatostatin-like immunoreactivity in the human foetus and spinal cord. Dev Brain Res 1987; 36: 63–73

28 Charnay Y, Paulin JA, Chayville JA, Dubois PM. Distribution of substance P like immunoreactivity in the spinal cord and dorsal root ganglia of the human foetus and infant. Neuroscience 1983; 10: 41–55

29 Fitzgerald M. The prenatal growth of fine diameter primary afferents into the rat spinal cord—a transganglionic study. J Comp Neurol 1987; 261: 98–104

30 Pignatelli D, Ribeiro-da-Silva A, Coimbra A. Postnatal maturation of primary afferent terminations in the substantia gelatinosa of the rat spinal cord. An electron microscope study. Brain Res 1989; 491: 33–44

31 Fitzgerald M. A physiological study of the prenatal development of cutaneous sensory inputs to dorsal horn cells in the rat. J Physiol 1991; 432: 473–482

32 Fitzgerald M. The development of activity evoked by fine diameter cutaneous fibres in the spinal cord of the newborn rat. Neurosci Lett 1988; 86: 161–166

33 Nussbaumer J-C, Yanagisawa M, Otsuka M. Pharmacological properties of a C-fibre response evoked by saphenous nerve stimulation in an isolated spinal cord-nerve preparation of the newborn rat. Br J Pharmacol 1989; 98: 373–382

34 Okado N, Kojima T. Ontogeny of the central nervous system: neurogenesis, fibre connection, synaptogenesis and myelination in the spinal cord. In: Prechtl HFR, ed. Continuity of Neural Functions from Prenatal to Postnatal Life. Clin Dev Med 1984; 94: 79–92

35 Bicknell HR, Beal JA. Axonal and dendritic development of substantia gelatinosa neurons in the lumbosacral spinal cord of the rat. J Comp Neurol 1984; 226: 508–522

36 Rizvi T, Wadha S, Bijlani V. Development of a spinal substrate for nociception. Pain 1987; (Suppl 4): 195

37 Fitzgerald M. The postnatal development of cutaneous afferent fibre input and receptive field organization in the rat dorsal horn. J Physiol 1985; 364: 1–18

38 Ekholm J. Postnatal changes in cutaneous reflexes and in the discharge pattern of cutaneous and articular sense organs. Acta Physiol Scand 1967; (Suppl); 297: 1–130

39 Charnay Y, Paulin C, Dray F, Dubois PM. Distribution of enkephalin in human foetus and infant spinal cord: an immunofluorescence study. J Comp Neurol 1985; 223: 415–423

40 Barr GA, Paredes W, Erickson KL, Zukin RS. κ-opioid receptor mediated analgesia in the developing rat. Dev Brain Res 1986; 29: 145–152

41 Zhang AZ, Pasternak GW. Ontogeny of opioid pharmacology and receptors: high and low affinity site differences. Eur J Pharmacol 1981; 73: 29–40

42 Charlton CG, Helke CJ. Ontogeny of substance P receptors in the rat spinal cord: quantitative changes in receptor number and differential expression in specific loci. Dev Brain Res 1986; 29: 81–91

43 Leong SK. Localizing the corticospinal neurons in neonatal, developing and mature albino rats. Brain Res 1983; 265: 1–9

44 Fitzgerald M. The development of descending brainstem control of spinal cord sensory processing. In: Hanson M, ed. Fetal and Neonatal Brainstem: Developmental and Clinical Issues. Cambridge: Cambridge University Press, 1991

45 Bregman BS. Development of serotonin immunoreactivity in the rat spinal cord and its plasticity after neonatal spinal cord lesions. Dev Brain Res 1987; 34: 245–263

46 Loizou LA. The postnatal ontogeny of monoamine-containing neurones in the central nervous system of the albino rat. Brain Res 1972; 40: 395–418

47 Commissiong JW. The development of catecholaminergic nerves in the spinal cord of the rat. II. Regional development. Dev Brain Res 1983; 11: 75–92

48 Fitzgerald M, Koltzenburg M. The functional development of descending inhibitory pathways in the dorsolateral funiculus of the newborn rat spinal cord. Dev Brain Res 1986; 24: 261–270

49 Thairu BK. Postnatal changes in the somaesthetic evoked potentials of the albino rat. Nature 1971; 231: 30–31

50 Klimach VJ, Cooke RWI. Maturation of the neonatal somatosensory evoked response in preterm infants. Dev Med Child Neurol 1988; 30: 208–214

51 Mrzljak L, Uylings HBM, Kostovic I, van Eden CG. Prenatal development of neurons in the human prefrontal cortex: a qualitative golgi study. J Comp Neurol 1988; 271: 355–386

52 Himes BT, Tessler A. Death of some DRG neurons and plasticity of others following sciatic nerve section in adult and neonatal rats. J Comp Neurol 1989; 284: 215–230

53 Fitzgerald M, Woolf CJ, Shortland P. Collateral sprouting of the central terminals of cutaneous primary afferent neurons in the rat spinal cord: pattern, morphology and influence of targets. J Comp Neurol 1990; 300: 2–17

54 Shortland P, Fitzgerald M. Functional connections formed by saphenous nerve terminal sprouts in the dorsal horn following neonatal sciatic nerve section. Eur J Neurosci (in press)

55 Fitzgerald M, Shortland P. The effect of neonatal peripheral nerve section on the somatodendritic growth of sensory projection cells in the rat spinal cord. Dev Brain Res 1988; 42: 129–136

56 Kaas JH, Merzenich MM, Killackey HP. The reorganization of somatosensory cortex following peripheral nerve damage in adult and developing mammals. Annu Rev Neurosci 1983; 6: 325–356

57 Killackey HP, Dawson DR. Expansion of the central hindpaw representation following fetal forelimb removal in the rat. Eur J Neurosci 1989; 1: 210–221

58 Chimelli L, Scaravilli F. Secondary transneuronal degeneration: cortical changes induced by peripheral nerve section in neonatal rats. Neurosci Lett 1985; 57: 57–63

British Medical Bulletin (1991) Vol. 47, No. 3, pp. 676–689
© The British Council 1991

Pain management in children

A Goldman, A R Lloyd-Thomas
Hospital for Sick Children, Great Ormond Street, London

Interest in the management and study of pain in children
has increased in recent years. A range of techniques
appropriate to children with different developmental levels
is now available for the assessment of various aspects of
childhood pain. A management plan can be developed
depending on the cause of pain and choosing from a
range of therapeutic techniques. It should take into
account both the physical and psychological aspects of
pain. Drugs form the mainstay of treatment of pain with a
clear physiological cause. Suitable drugs are now available
but inexperience and myths may still result in reluctance to
use appropriate strong analgesics in children. Postoperative pain control and the analgesic needs of neonates
have been particularly neglected areas. Management can
be dramatically improved by increasing staff sensitivity and
the use of an integrated programme of drugs, physical
techniques and psychological approaches.

After many years of neglect, both in clinical practice and research,
interest in pain in children is increasing. This is important for the
children themselves and also because it is becoming clear that pain
suffered in childhood, the physical and emotional memories of it
and the coping strategies developed can influence a person's
responses to pain throughout their lives.

The management of pain in children has tended to be frag-
mented. Post-operative pain management has been the province
of anaesthetists and pain from procedures and specific diseases has
been addressed by hospital specialists; with cancer tackled by paediatric oncologists, sickle cell disease by haematologists and recurrent abdominal pain being the province of general paediatricians.
The role of psychologists, physiotherapists and other paramedical

personnel has been quite variable and less prominent in this country than the USA. The recent interest in childhood pain has been accompanied by efforts to establish approaches which cross some of these boundaries and offer the patient the benefits of a team approach.[1] There is evidence from adult practice that the creation of a specialized pain control team dramatically improves the management of post-operative pain.[2] In paediatrics a dedicated team has the potential to bring together the medical, anaesthetic and psychosocial skills needed to address the range of situations where pain is a problem. They also have a role in research and in education of patients, parents, nurses and doctors.

CAUSES

A rigid classification of the causes of pain in children is difficult. It can be helpful to consider pain experiences as acute, chronic or recurrent and also to identify both the psychological and physical components in any pain situation. Acute pains include those caused by a clear tissue damaging stimulus such as trauma or burns or diseases such as sickle cell crises or cancer. A large group of children have acute pain problems associated with medical intervention, such as post surgery, with repeated venepuncture, investigations or therapeutic injections. Chronic pain may be produced by prolonged diseases such as arthritis or pains which exist beyond the expected time for healing. The chronic persistent pains such as back aches, so frequent in adults, are uncommon in children, but recurrent episodic pains such as headaches, abdominal or limb pain in otherwise healthy children do occur quite commonly and can prove frustrating diagnostic and management problems.

PAIN ASSESSMENT

The undertreatment of pain in children has been attributed in part to the difficulty of assessing and measuring children's pain. This challenge has been the focus of considerable progress recently. Although the assessment of pain in children is more difficult than adults there are now a number of practical methods available and these have been reviewed in detail.[3,4] Much of the work so far has been part of research projects particularly in acute pain. The routine use of pain assessment techniques in the clinical setting, particularly for children with chronic pain, still needs to be developed.

Methods for assessing pain in infants and children can be physiological, behavioural or subjective.

A number of physiological parameters have been investigated as measures of pain severity. The theoretical advantages are that they can provide an objective result and can be used in preverbal children. These are counterbalanced by the difficulty of getting consistent results and of knowing whether the responses and changes initiated by the noxious stimulus actually correlate directly with pain. In neonates cardiovascular changes, oxygen saturation or tension, palmar sweating and hormonal and metabolic changes have been used as measures reflecting stress following acute pain and efforts have been made to correlate these with the neonates behavioural state.[5]

Another approach to pain measurement is by observations of infants' and children's behaviour in response to a painful stimulus. Care is needed to select well-defined behaviours, to minimize error between observers and to choose an appropriate time period for observations. Most work to date has been in a research setting and with acute pain. In infants changes in facial expressions, body movement and cry patterns occur with painful stress but the reactions are complex and vary with age and prior state of arousal and behaviour. In older children a number of scales to evaluate the pain of invasive medical procedures have been developed and validated. The procedural behaviour rating scale—revised (PBRS-r)[6,7] was developed for paediatric oncology procedures originally and the Children's Hospital of Eastern Ontario Pain Scale (CHEOPS)[8] for assessing post-operative pain. These can be useful as part of a pain-relieving programme both as research tools and for individual children.

The most valuable information about a child's pain is obtained by assessing their subjective experience. If an appropriate technique is used, children as young as three years old can provide information about their pain. Detailed pain questionnaires which look at the broad picture of pain including the history, previous pain experience and affective aspects of the pain as well as intensity are available such as the Varni-Thompson Paediatric Pain Questionnaire (VTPPQ)[9] and the Children's Comprehensive Pain Questionnaire (CCPQ).[3] These are particularly valuable when assessing children with chronic and recurrent pains. A number of measures for pain intensity are available. Those developed for adults such as visual analogue scales and numerical scales can be used by older children and adolescents but more concrete variations of these are needed for younger children. Graded scales of facial expressions, either drawings[10] or photographs[11,12] are available. The colour tool developed by Eland is an imaginative technique where children construct their own pain scale using eight different coloured crayons which they grade from 'no hurt at all' to 'worst hurt' and they can use them to colour in a body outline.[13,14] Hester's Poker Chip Tool helps children quantify their pain by visualizing it as pieces of hurt which they can then grade from one to four.[15]

Detailed assessment of a child in pain is important and is a step towards diagnosing the cause and nature of the pain so that an effective plan of management can be developed. Since a wide range of measurement tools are now available the method used needs to be chosen carefully and often a combination will be most successful. The tests need to reflect the child's age and cognitive development. An appropriate subjective method is preferable but in babies and infants behavioural and physiological techniques will have to be relied on. The clinical situation will influence one's choice so that for chronic and recurrent pains detailed questionnaires covering broad aspects may be needed whereas for acute pain information about severity and distribution of pain may be more relevant.

TREATMENT APPROACHES

Drugs

Drugs form the mainstay of treatment of pain with a clear physiological cause. Pharmaceutical development has afforded a wide range of analgesic drugs. Our failure to adequately control pain results not from lack of suitable drugs but our own inability to use them properly. Our current practice is based upon pain relief, but there is increasing evidence that pathological pain stimuli induce both peripheral and central excitability thereby exaggerating pain transmission from surrounding areas.[16] Our attention should, perhaps, be directed to pain prevention by appropriate medication before the adverse stimulus (pre-emptive analgesia).[17]

Peripheral nociceptor sensitization may be caused by chemicals released by damaged tissue (bradykinin, histamine, substance P, leukotrienes and prostaglandins) which may be attenuated by anti-inflammatory drugs. Central sensitization occurs as a result of C fibre afferents changing the excitability of dorsal horn neurones which may respond to opioids. A combined approach using both types of drugs may be appropriate.

Mild analgesics

Paracetamol is widely used for discomfort in children. It is only a weak inhibitor of general prostaglandin synthesis but is often effective for mild pain. The use of aspirin in children is precluded by its association with Reye's syndrome. In children with disseminated malignancy with bone marrow involvement aspirin is also to be avoided because of its adverse effects on platelets in children whose count is already low. However it continues to have an important role in the treatment of inflammation and pain in juvenile chronic arthritis.

Non steroid anti-inflammatory agents (NSAIDs)

These are useful for pains of inflammatory origin such as juvenile chronic arthritis and children with bony metastases whose platelet counts are adequate. All NSAIDs can cause gastritis and if used for long periods renal and hepatic function should be monitored. Experience with NSAIDs for surgery in children has been limited to tonsillectomy and dental extraction with conflicting results between studies in the quality of analgesia achieved and degree of opioid sparing. Work in adults suggests that NSAIDs will be more effective in surgery with significant peripheral tissue injury (e.g. orthopaedic surgery) provided they are started before the operation. They appear to work better in lower abdominal surgery rather than upper abdominal operations where they have little beneficial action.

It is not possible to predict to which of the NSAIDs a child's pain will respond best and choice may also be influenced by which are available as elixirs or long acting preparations. NSAIDs are known to exhibit a poor dose response relationship and titration of the dose against individual patient response rather than fixed dose regimens may be the key to success with these drugs.

Moderate analgesics

Mild opioids such as codeine can be used for pain which is not responsive to mild analgesics. Paracetamol can be used in combination with codeine (ratio 10:1 Formulix Cilag) for moderate pain, such as that associated with minor surgery when regional or peripheral blocks wear off. Mild opioids have the same potential side effects as strong opioids, described below, but in practice are well tolerated. For the child with pain of progressive malignancy they form a useful stepping stone from mild analgesics to strong opioids.

Strong opioid analgesics

There is now a wide range of pure and partial agonists available but morphine remains the standard against which all are judged. Experience has been gained with morphine in children, in whom it is an effective analgesic. The most common uses of strong opioids are in the care of post-operative patients and for children with progressive malignant disease or other terminal illnesses which are described in more detail below. Many myths and fears still persist both in the public and among professionals which prevent appropriate use of opioids. Successful introduction of these drugs often depends on tackling these concerns.

PSYCHOLOGICAL MANAGEMENT

Psychological approaches should not be reserved for children whose pain has no clear pathological cause. Fear, anxiety and stress contribute to all painful experiences and manoeuvres to reduce them should form part of a comprehensive management plan. A range of techniques are available.

Preparation has a vital role in the care of children. Hospitals can be strange and frightening and medical interventions may seem arbitrary and endless. Younger children who are not yet able to think logically easily misinterpret events, find difficulty in distinguishing cause and effect and can build up terrifying and bewildering fantasies. At the simplest level the child can be given information about the hospital and procedures, what is being done and how he might feel, both before and during an admission. Parents should be involved and included as they provide a child's greatest sense of security. There are many other preparations which have been used to help children feel some sense of control and understanding. Many are instigated by trained play specialists and include the use of books, doll play, hospital toys and art.[18]

Distraction and hypnosis can be useful tools in pain management. The response to a noxious stimulus is reduced when concentration is focused elsewhere. Many parents use distraction with children routinely without thinking about it and will, for example, initiate a new activity with a child if they fall and hurt themselves. Parents can be encouraged and shown effective ways to use distraction in clinical situations. The activity needs to be of sufficient interest and age appropriate such as blowing bubbles for a young child or using computer games for school age children during a venepuncture.

The nature of hypnotic analgesia is not well understood but hypnosis has been used successfully to help children in a number of different pain situations. It has been used with children during procedures,[19] those with sickle cell disease,[20] migraine[21] and cancer.[22] Children are excellent subjects for hypnosis and imagery techniques which they enjoy and there are no unpleasant side-effects. Parents can learn to help and both they and the children benefit from this sense of control. A therapist with skill and imagination can work with the children helping them to get pain relief as they identify in adventures with favourite television or cartoon heroes, by making journeys in magical lands or by learning to 'turn off' painful parts of their body.

Behavioural approaches such as desensitization and positive reinforcement techniques can be used to counteract unhelpful learned responses to both acute and recurrent pain problems. Counselling for the child or family may be needed where dysfunction or reactions to critical life events appear to be contributing significantly, especially in chronic and recurrent pain situations.

POST-OPERATIVE ANALGESIA

The most common analgesic prescription following surgery continues to be intermittent, as required, intramuscular injections of a narcotic, despite the knowledge that this technique results in poor control of pain. Doctors are wary of overprescribing opioids and this mode of prescription has the superficial attraction of being simple to write so that only the minimum dosage will be given. However, it delegates responsibility for administration to others and they may be inexperienced in pain assessment, they are often inappropriately worried by the risk of side-effects or causing addiction and are therefore reluctant to medicate patients adequately. Surveys of this technique in children show that they receive fewer, less frequent and smaller doses of narcotics in comparison with adults, whilst minor analgesics are used much earlier in the postoperative course.[23] The control of post-operative pain in children remains poor.[24] It requires an integrated approach of drugs, usually opioids, local anaesthetics and sensitivity of staff to concerns about pain in children and parents.

The advantage of giving morphine by infusion is that it can be titrated readily against patient response to provide smooth analgesia impossible to achieve with 'prn' intramuscular injection (10–30 mcg/kg/h, loading dose 100–200 mcg/kg top up dose if required four hourly 50–100 mcg/kg). Periods of arterial oxygen desaturation have been described in adults during REM sleep using this technique and this is currently being investigated in children. The children must be under regular nursing observation.

The partial agonists, meptazinol (1 mg/kg), nalbuphine (0.15– 0.3 mg/kg) and buprenorphine (parenteral 3–6 mcg/kg, sublingual 5–7 mcg/kg) have all been investigated in children and found to be satisfactory but they represent little advantage over morphine in children. The sublingual route and dose formulation of buprenorphine (220 mcg tablets) makes it impractical for most children.

Patient controlled analgesia has been shown to have considerable advantages in adult practice and this technique can be offered to children older than 8 years. Using morphine, a background infusion (5 mcg/kg/h) combined with patient controlled boluses (10 mcg/kg) and a lockout interval of 10–15 minutes but subject to a maximum of 500 mcg/kg in any 4 hour period, has been found to be satisfactory in this hospital. At present, most infusion devices do not have control programmes designed to give the small doses required by children and development of these are needed before patient controlled analgesia can expand to younger children.

Segmental analgesia can be produced by giving narcotics into the cerebrospinal fluid or in the extradural space. Optimal analgesia may be provided by the combination of extradural local anaesthetics, to attenuate pain transmission and extradural opioids, to prevent C fibre excitation, given before the onset of pain.

For major surgery, a programme of extradural analgesia has been introduced at this hospital. After intra-operation use (bupivacaine 0.25% plain as required, diamorphine single bolus at start of surgery 50 mcg/kg), an infusion of 0.125% bupivacaine (0.125% given at 0.2 ml/kg/h) combined with diamorphine (5 mcg/kg/h) given by continuous infusion, has provided excellent analgesia to children ranging from 2 months to adolescence.

Accurate siting of the catheter adjacent to the dermatomes to be blocked is essential. The hazard of delayed respiratory depression with extradural narcotics is equally important in children as in adults. For this reason we confine this technique to areas with a high nurse to patient ratio, and forbid narcotics by any other route.

Local anaesthesia used for wound infiltration, nerve blocks, plexus blocks and regional blocks is important in providing pain relief for children following surgery. Most minor surgery in children is performed on a day care basis and this is not possible without good local anaesthetic techniques providing pain relief, without the nausea and vomiting associated with narcotics. Bupivacaine is the most popular choice in paediatric local analgesia as it has a long duration of action and a good safety record. Plain bupivacaine (0.25%) is satisfactory for most blocks in children. The dose is determined by the site of the block, subject to a maximum dose of 3 mg/kg.

CANCER PAIN

For the child with progressive malignant disease when pain is no longer relieved by weaker analgesics strong opioids should be used. For parents there is often an emotional hurdle in admitting their child's disease has progressed to the extent of needing opioids. This may need to be explored before they will tolerate giving the drugs. Inappropriate concerns of hastening the child's death, of addiction and fears of side effects will often need to be clarified with medical and nursing staff.

Although opioids decrease the respiratory response to hypoxia and hypercapnia there appears to be a wide margin between the doses required for analgesia and those causing respiratory failure. Respiratory depression is uncommon in patients receiving opioids for pain due to cancer and appears to be no more common in children above the age of 3 months old than in adults with comparable plasma opioid levels.[25] Confusion still arises between physical dependence and psychological addiction to opioids. Physiological dependence will develop following regular administration of opioids over one or two weeks but this rarely presents a clinical problem. If a child's pain and therefore their analgesic needs decrease, for example after radiotherapy to a bony metastasis, then symptoms of withdrawal can be avoided by gradually decreasing the dose of opioids over a number of days. There is no evidence that appropriate administration of opioids for pain produces psychological addiction.

In practice the side effects of clinical concern in children on opioids for chronic pain are initial sedation and constipation. Sedation is common in children particularly over the first two days of using a strong opioid but it wears off. It is very important to warn parents about this as otherwise they may attribute the child's drowsiness to rapid disease progression and may fear their imminent death. Constipation is also common and can be troublesome if adequate laxatives are not given routinely. Regular lactulose is often sufficient and is well tolerated by children but, if not, oral stimulant laxatives or rectal preparations should be introduced. Nausea attributable to opioids appears to be rare. Overt dysphoria is also rare in children, although some report vivid nightmares. Pruritis is uncommon and may respond to antihistamines. Occasionally it can be intolerable and alternative opioid preparations may be better tolerated. The active metabolite of morphine is excreted renally and in patients with renal impairment care must be taken with the dose and frequency of administration of strong opioids to avoid overdose.

The route of choice for opioids for children with chronic pain is oral. Morphine is available in preparations active over 3–4 hours and also in slow release form, (MST Contin) active over 12 hours. The advantage to children of the less frequent medication is considerable. The theoretical disadvantage is lack of flexibility in dose variation but this can be overcome by providing patients with a short acting morphine preparation to use whilst gradually increasing the dose to give full analgesia and also for breakthrough pain. Patients vary in the dose of opioids required to produce analgesia and the dose should be titrated to produce the required clinical effect. Initial recommended doses of MST for children who have pain which has been unresponsive to codeine are 1 mg/kg/dose twice daily.[26] For 4-hourly oral morphine 0.3 mg/kg/dose is suggested.

Nausea and vomiting, decreased level of consciousness, inability to swallow or occasionally flat refusal to take oral medication may make it necessary to find an alternative route. Rectal preparations of morphine and the longer acting oxycodone are available. For some patients and staff they are not an attractive choice but they can be useful, particularly in children who are no longer conscious and within the last hours before death. The most convenient alternative to the oral route is a continuous subcutaneous infusion. Drugs can be delivered by a small portable syringe driver attached to a narrow gauge needle, sited on the abdominal wall, upper arm or leg. The syringe containing drugs can be replaced every 24 hours and parents can be taught how to do this. If the child has a permanent indwelling intravenous catheter, such as a Hickman, then this can be used conveniently for a continuous infusion, but the disadvantage of the intravenous route is that tolerance builds up rapidly and escalation to much higher doses may be needed.

Pain is a great fear for parents and older children with cancer and a comprehensive management plan should be developed for each individual patient. Depending on the situation opioid drugs can be used with NSAIDs, anticonvulsants and antidepressants for neuropathic pain, palliative radiation, regional anaesthetic techniques and psychological approaches. Regular review and support by experienced staff enable most children to be managed comfortably at home if that is the family's wish.[27]

NEONATES

Newborn babies are also subjected to painful procedures especially if they require surgery or intensive care. In adults or older children there would be no doubt that this treatment may result in pain but generous interpretation of early work led many practitioners to suggest that neonates could not feel pain.[28,29] This has been compounded by lack of knowledge and fear of side effects of opioid analgesics in neonates with the result that they have been withheld.

Recent evidence suggests that pain transmission does occur in neonates and the outcome of surgery may be improved by giving analgesics.[5,30] Attention should therefore be directed to the management of pain in neonates, either by the use of local anaesthetics or narcotics, although the potential hazards of the latter should not be underestimated. The side-effects of opioids, particularly respiratory depression, are seen more frequently in new born infants.[31] This increased sensitivity arises from altered pharmacokinetics secondary to immature excretory pathways[32] increased permeability of the immature blood-brain barrier increased concentrations of endogenous opioids in blood and cerebrospinal fluid[33] and changes in the proportion of Mu-1 and Mu-2 receptors in the developing brain.[34]

Individual neonates show wide variability in their degree of sensitivity to opioids and this difference is not predictable on clinical grounds. In neonates receiving mechanical ventilation both morphine (5–10 mcg/kg/h) or fentanyl (2–4 mcg/kg/h) given by infusion have been used successfully with the latter being the best choice for those at risk of pulmonary hypertension. When compared with adults, the neonatal elimination half-life for both drugs is prolonged and excretion is further delayed in critically ill babies, which may result in drug accumulating. The infusion must be titrated against patient response and terminated well in advance of weaning from mechanical ventilation. Newer synthetic narcotics such as sufentanil and alfentanil may prove to be useful in this age group.

The pain of surgery in neonates can also be managed using local anaesthetics, although care with dosage is required as they are more susceptible to local anaesthetic toxicity.[35] Bupivacaine plain (0.25% maximum dose 2 mg/kg) has a long duration of action and a good safety record in this age group. Stronger solutions are not required in neonates as myelination is not complete. All local anaesthetic techniques such as wound infiltration, peripheral nerve blocks, plexus blocks or extradural blocks can be used for neonates. Unfortunately analgesia is still rarely given for circumcision, one of the most common surgical operations performed in neonates.

PAINFUL PROCEDURES

A eutectic mixture of lignocaine-prilocaine cream (EMLA) applied to the skin 90 minutes before venepuncture markedly reduces the pain of blood sampling and venous cannulation.[36] It has also been used recently in a double blind trial for pain associated with lumbar punctures.[37] Although a beneficial effect of EMLA cream was demonstrated it also showed the favourable effect of a placebo. In the newborn prilocaine can be absorbed and result in methaemaglobinaemia. Neonates are particularly susceptible because of low levels of the enzyme methaemaglobin reductase. Care needs to be taken to limit the quantity and duration of application of EMLA especially in preterm infants.

Behavioural techniques have a significant role to play in painful procedures. Distraction and hypnosis have been used for venepuncture, lumbar punctures and bone marrow aspirates.

REFERENCES

1 Berde C, Sethna NF, Masek B, Fosburg M, Rocklin S. Pediatric Pain Clinics: Recommendations for their Development. Pediatrician 1989; 16: 94–102
2 Ready LB, Oden R, Chadwick HS et al. Development of an anesthesiology-based post-operative pain management service. Anesthesiology 1988; 68: 101–106

3 McGrath PA. Pain in Children: nature, assessment and treatment. Guilford: Guilford Press, 1990
4 McGrath PJ, Unruh A. Pain in Children. Amsterdam: Elsevier, 1987
5 Anand KJS, Hickey PR. N Engl J Med 1987; 317: 1321–1329
6 Katz ER, Kellerman J, Siegel SE. Behavioural distress in children with cancer undergoing medical procedures: Developmental considerations. J Consult Clin Psychol 1980; 48: 356–365
7 Katz ER, Kellerman J, Siegel SE. Anxiety as an affective focus in the clinical study of acute behavioral distress: A reply to Shacham and Daut. J Consult Clin Psychol 1981; 49: 470–471
8 McGrath PJ, Johnson G, Goodman JT, Schillinger J, Dunn J, Chapman J. The CHEOPS: a behavioral scale to measure post operative pain in children. In: Fields HL, Dubner R, Cervero F, eds. Advances in Pain Research and Therapy. New York: Raven Press, 1985
9 Varni JW, Thompson KL, Hanson V. The Varni/Thompson Pediatric Pain Questionnaire: 1. Chronic muscolo-skeletal pain in juvenile rheumatoid arthritis. Pain 1987; 28: 27–38
10 McGrath PA, de Veber LL, Hearn MT. Multidimensional pain assessment in children. In: Fields HL, Dubner R, Cervero F, eds. Advances in Pain Research and Therapy. New York: Raven Press, 1985
11 Beyer J, Aradine C. Content validity of an instrument to measure young children's perceptions of the intensity of their pain. J Pediatr Nurs 1986; 1: 386–395
12 Beyer J, Aradine C. Patterns of pediatric pain intensity: A methodological investigation of a self-report scale. Clin J Pain 1987; 3: 130–141
13 Eland JM, Anderson JE. The experience of pain in children. In: Jacox AK ed. Pain: A source book for nurses and other health professionals. Boston: Little Brown, 1977
14 Eland JM. Minimising injection pain associated with prekindergarten immunizations. Issues Compr Pediatr Nurs 1982; 5: 361–372
15 Hester NO. The preoperational child's reaction to immunisation. Nurs Res 1979; 28: 250–254
16 Fitzgerald M, Millard C, McIntosh N. Cutaneous hyper-sensitivity following peripheral tissue damage in newborn infants and its reversal with topical anaesthesia. Pain 1989; 39: 31–36
17 Woolf CJ. Recent advances in the pathophysiology of acute pain. Br J Anaesth 1989; 63: 139–146
18 Peterson G. Let the children play. Nursing 1989; 3: 22–25
19 Zeltzer L, LeBaron S. Hypnosis and nonhypnotic techniques for reduction of pain and anxiety during painful procedures in children and adolescents with cancer. J Pediatr 1982; 101: 1032–1035
20 Zeltzer L, Dash J, Holland JP. Hypnotically induced pain control in sickle cell anemia. Pediatrics 1979; 64: 533–536
21 Olness K, MacDonald J. Self-hypnosis and biofeedback in the management of juvenile migraine. J Dev Behav Pediatr 1981; 2: 168–170
22 Hilgard JR, LeBaron S. Hypnotherapy of Pain in Children with Cancer. William Kaufmann, 1984
23 Schechter NL, Allen DA, Hanson K. Status of paediatric pain control: A comparison of hospital analgesic usage in children and adults. Paediatrics 1986; 77: 11–15
24 Mather L, Mackie J. The incidence of post-operative pain in children. Pain 1983; 15: 271–292
25 Shannon M, Berde C. Pharmacologic management of pain in children and adolescents. Pediatr Clin N Am 1989; 36: 855–872
26 Goldman A, Bowman A. The role of oral controlled release morphine for pain relief in children with cancer. Palliat Med 1990; 4: 279–285

27 Goldman A, Beardsmore S, Hunt J. Palliative care for children with cancer—home, hospital or hospice. Arch Dis Child 1990; 65: 641–643
28 McGraw MD. The neuromuscular maturation of the human infant. New York: Columbia University Press, 1943
29 Tilney F, Rossett J. The value of brain lipoids as an index of brain development. Bull Neurol Inst New York, 1931; 1: 28–71
30 Anand KJS, Sippell WG, Aynsley-Green A. Randomised trial of fentanyl anaesthesia in preterm babies undergoing surgery: effects on the stress response. Lancet 1987; i: 62–66
31 Purcell-Jones G, Dormon F, Sumner E. The use of opioids in neonates. A retrospective study of 933 cases. Anaesthesia 1987; 42: 1316–1320
32 Koren G, Butt W, Chinyanga, Soldin S, Tan YK, Pape K. Postoperative morphine infusion in newborn infants: assessment of disposition characteristics and safety. J Paediatr 1985; 107: 963–967
33 Orlowski JP. Cerebrospinal fluid endorphins and the infant apnoea syndrome. Paediatrics 1986; 78: 233–237
34 Leslie FM, Tso S, Harlbutt DE. Differential appearance of opiate receptor subtypes in neonatal rat brain. Life Sciences 1982; 31: 1393–1396
35 Lloyd-Thomas AR. Pain management in paediatric patients. Br J Anaesth 1990; 64: 85–104
36 Wahstedt C, Kollberg H, Moller C, Uppfeldt A. Lignocaine—Prilocaine cream reduces venepuncture pain. Lancet 1984; 106
37 Kapelushnik J, Koren G, Solh H, Greenberg M, DeVeber L. Evaluating the efficacy of EMLA in alleviating pain associated with lumbar puncture; comparison of open and double-blinded protocols in children. Pain 1990; 42: 31–34

British Medical Bulletin (1991) Vol. 47, No. 3, pp. 690–702
© The British Council 1991

Mechanisms of the analgesic actions of opiates and opioids

A H Dickenson
Department of Pharmacology, University College, London, UK

It is now clear that there are three sub-types of the opiate receptor, mu, delta and kappa. Evidence for differential roles of these sub-types in pain modulation is accumulating since the advent of relatively selective agonists and more recently, antagonists for the three receptors. The actions of opioids in the spinal cord is reasonably well understood and there is increasing knowledge of supraspinal sites of action, peripheral analgesic effects in inflammatory states and in the interactions between opioid and non-opioid systems at spinal levels, which may start to explain some of the clinical states with altered opioid sensitivity.

The discovery of the opioid receptor followed by the isolation and identification of the endogenous opioid peptides has at present had little impact on the treatment of pain. It is to be hoped that this will alter in the not too distant future. However it has already caused an enormous advance in our understanding of the mechanisms of action of opioids in the production of analgesia and insights into the roles of peptides in central nervous function—an area which now embraces a large number of putative non-opioid peptide transmitters (Fig. 1).

The endogenous opioids, the enkephalins, dynorphins and endorphin family are all peptide in nature and there is a reasonable correspondence between these three main families of opioid peptides and the three receptors they act on.[1] However, no endogenous opioid is specific for any one receptor. The susceptibility of the opioids to peptidase degradation together with the lack of selectivity for the receptor subtypes has lead to the synthesis of stable

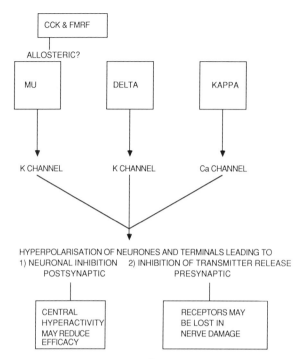

Fig. 1 The three main opioid receptor subtypes and their effector mechanisms together with the interactions between the opioid and other systems which may interfere with analgesia.

analogues some of which have proved to be useful research tools for probing receptor function. It is to be hoped that these derivatives will lead to clinically useful agents, based on the premise that drugs which act on receptors other than the morphine site could lack the morphine like side effects which can cause problems in man. Table 1 lists the current state of knowledge of opioid receptors and their ligands.

The three main families of opioids are all derived from different precursers so that the propeptides for the endorphins, enkephalins and the dynorphins are quite separate. Recently detection of the messenger RNA for the propeptides have allowed the neurones containing the different opioids to be unequivocally identified and the levels of mRNA serve as a measure of opioid peptide synthesis under various conditions. There are discrepancies between the receptors and ligands in some areas of the body, a prime example being a high level of mu opioid receptors in the spinal cord but

Table 1 Opioid receptors and their ligands

Receptor	Mu	Delta	Kappa
Endogenous ligands	β-endorphin	met-enkephalin	dynorphins
	dermorphin	leu-enkephalin	
	metorphamide		
Synthetic ligands	morphine	DPDPE	U50488H
	fentanyl	DTLET	U69893
	methadone*	DSTBULET	PD117302
	DAGOL		Pentazocine
Antagonists	naloxone	naloxone	naloxone
	(low dose)	(med. dose)	(high dose)
	β-FNA	ICI174864	nor-BNI

*Most clinically used opioids are predominantly mu agonists.
DAGOL, DPDPE, DTLET and DSTBULET are all peptide analogues based on enkephalin. (see Refs 1,15,17,23,26)
U50488H, U69893 and PD117302 are non-peptide kappa agonists and are active systematically. (see Refs 1,20,22,44)
β-FNA is β-funaltrexamine, an irreversible antagonist.
nor-BNI- is nor-binaltorphimine.

no obvious endogenous opioid for this receptor in this region. This may reflect yet unknown endogenous opioids or deficiencies in the anatomical techniques. There is intriguing evidence that morphine itself may be endogenous since the plant synthetic pathway is present in the mammal and there are regional differences in the levels of traces of morphine in the CNS.[2]

IONIC EFFECTS OF THE OPIOIDS

The three opioid receptor subtypes all produce primary inhibitory effects following receptor activation.[3-5] There are a number of excitatory or facilitatory effects of opioids all of which can nevertheless be explained on the basis of inhibition being the only result of opioid receptor activation. The activation of mu and delta receptors by a variety of ligands produce an opening of K^+ channels, not directly, but via either cyclic AMP and/or G protein intermediaries. The net result of this action on a neurone would be hyperpolarisation and a reduction in firing whereas at a terminal the effect would be a reduced Ca^{2+} influx and inhibition of transmitter release. If the inhibited cell was itself an inhibitory neurone the next cell in the line would be released from inhibition and so excited, by a primary opioid hyperpolarizing effect, an example of disinhibition. Opioid disinhibitions of this nature have been observed in the substantia gelatinosa of the spinal cord and in the hippocampus. Kappa opioids appear to act by closing Ca^{2+} channels. Thus while the mu and delta receptors have similar modes of action, the kappa receptor differs from the others, not only in terms of primary mechanism of action but also in some functional consequences of its activation.

There are some interesting developmental differences in the ontogeny of these opioid receptors such that the mu and kappa receptors arrive early in development of the CNS with the delta receptor appearing later but the kappa receptors in spinal areas can alter as the animal ages, maybe due to subtypes of the receptors developing.[6]

SPINAL ANALGESIA

The spinal cord is an important site in the production of analgesia as has been clearly shown by the demonstration of opioid inhibition of nociceptive neurones in spinal animals, direct analgesia following epidural and intrathecal opioids in animals and then subsequently in man.[7,8] There have been considerable efforts devoted to the study of opioid receptor subtypes in the spinal cord, using both electrophysiological and behavioural approaches. There is now a reasonable consensus regarding the relative roles of the mu and delta receptors but sharp disagreement on the kappa receptor at this level. The recent studies on the spinal opioid systems have started to address the extent of plasticity in opioid spinal function, with indications that opioid activity and function are not immutable, even to the extent of opioid peptide genes being activated by particular stimuli.

The advent of selective ligands has allowed the location and relative distribution of opioid receptor subtypes to be gauged. The highest levels of opioid receptors in the spinal cord are around the C-fibre terminal zones in lamina 1 and the substantia gelatinosa although smaller amounts are found in deeper layers. The best current estimates suggest that the mu receptor forms 70%, the delta 24% and the kappa 6% of the total opioid sites in the rat spinal cord. The proportions of pre- and postsynaptic sites varies for the subtypes estimated from drops in levels after rhizotomy (up to 70%).[9] There may be marked species differences, for example kappa levels appear higher in mouse and guinea pig. A presynaptic action of opioids has been demonstrated for mu and delta but not kappa agonists on the basis of a reduced release of the primary afferent transmitters present in C-fibres. The expected axo-axonic morphological basis for this has not been seen suggesting that there may be non-synaptic actions of opioids acting from afar.

The association of opioid receptors with C but not large A fibre terminals allows for the observed selective effects of spinal opioids on noxious evoked activity.[7,10] The postsynaptic actions of opioids are difficult to reconcile with their specificity of action since any direct hyperpolarization of a cell soma would inhibit all responses of the cell which would include the innocuous inputs onto convergent or multireceptive cells. However, many of the opioid receptors in the substantia gelatinosa could be on the dendrites of the deep cells penetrating into the C-fibre terminal zone; inhibitory effects here would also be selective. Another possibility is based on the observation of substantia gelatinosa cells being facilitated by opioids after many different routes of administration. This appears to be via $GABA_A$ mediated disinhibition of interneurones as has been observed in the hippocampus.[3] If these disinhibited cells fed onto the output cells they would be an additional source of inhibition. Whatever the case these different mechanisms will have overall similar final effects but pathological damage to the afferents will remove the presynaptic receptors on the terminals which has relevance to the treatment by opioids of neuropathic pain.

The ED_{50}'s of mu and delta opioids are similar in range but the most potent opioids are the mu ligands dermorphin, a natural peptide isolated from frog skin but found in the mammalian CNS,[11] and DAGOL, a modified version of enkephalin.[12] Their potencies presumably reflect the large number of mu opioid sites. The potency of DAGOL may be the reason for its relative lack of tolerance compared to less potent mu opioids since fewer receptors will need to be activated.[13] Relevant to the remarkable potency of the peptides after spinal application and of great importance to the clinical selection of opioid dose for spinal analgesia is the clear inverse relationship between lipophilicity and potency for a range of synthetic opioids.[14] This is probably due to non-specific binding in lipid rich fibre tracts capping the cord or vascular redistribution reducing the dose of opioid reaching the receptors in the gelatinosa. Interestingly a difference between the mu and delta receptors is that the lowest doses of mu opioids enhance C fibre activity with inhibitions taking over as the dose is increased.[10–12] This may be due to presynaptic autoreceptors or actions on terminal excitability and this mild increase in C fibre activity could explain the itching around the extremities of the spinal opioid injection seen in man. The use of antagonists for the mu and delta receptors has demonstrated their independence of action at the spinal level[15] and both receptors are effective in all tests of anti-nociception with the exception of visceral chemical stimuli where delta are less effective.[16] Since delta opioids dramatically reduce responses to cutaneous algogens this difference is likely to result from the origins of the stimulus not the nature of the stimulus itself.[17]

In the case of the kappa receptor the status of this receptor subtype as a mediator of spinal antinociception cannot yet be fully ascertained. Early behavioural studies using dynorphin itself can be disregarded due to the paralysis caused by the peptide.[18] Sub-sequent studies with synthetic ligands have in a minority of cases shown clear cut analgesia but many others have seen no effect or have had to reduce the stimulus intensity or pick certain modalities to reveal effects.[19,20] Electrophysiological studies have shown exci-tations as well as inhibitions after spinal application with only the highest doses producing inhibitions.[21] These inhibitions are insen-sitive to the kappa antagonist nor binaltorphamine. Studies where kappa analgesia has been reported need to be repeated to gauge effects of the antagonist. A few studies have suggested that higher doses of naloxone are needed to reverse kappa effects compared to mu[20] but it has still not been shown unequivocally that kappa ligands act via the kappa receptor and not on mu or other recep-tors. These disparate results are possibly due to the very low levels of spinal kappa receptors in the rat but kappa opioids have been reported to cause hyperalgesia in the guinea pig which has reason-able levels of spinal kappa opioid receptors.

It is interesting to note that the lack of a clear antinociceptive effect of spinal kappa opioids seen in electrophysiological and behavioural studies contrast with clear reversible kappa antinoc-iception seen in younger animals by the same groups.[22] Since a number of electrophysiological studies have shown obvious kappa effects in newborn animals it is quite possible that there are post natal changes in the kappa receptor with the adult version of the receptor being poorly associated with antinociception. There might be subtypes of the mu receptor but the evidence so far hinges on the use of one antagonist and needs to be verified.

A novel approach to the production of analgesia via the delta receptor is the synthesis of peptidase inhibitors of which, kelator-phan, a mixed peptidase inhibitor affords almost complete protec-tion to the enkephalins.[23,24] The spinal application of the inhibitor produces a reduction of nociceptive responses of cells,[24] with the pool of enkephalins likely to be derived from both a segmental release and from descending pathways activated by the stimulus. The inhibitions are reversed by a selective delta antagonist. Similar effects have been seen with another peptidase inhibitor in behavioural studies.

SUPRASPINAL ANALGESIA

At supraspinal sites the interactions between opioid receptor subtypes and neural substrates in different areas of the brainstem and midbrain has been well mapped in terms of location of effective opioid sites although the mechanisms of analgesia remain hazy. It is clearly established that a series of sites in the medial brain stem around the area of the nucleus raphe magnus and running up to periaqueductal and periventricular grey areas subserve morphine analgesia as based on microinjection studies and the ability of naloxone locally applied to reduce the effects of systemic morphine.[25] There is good evidence that mu and delta receptors are effective in eliciting analgesia at brain stem sites (kappa have not been widely tested) but after intraventricular administration the mu receptor can explain all the analgesia in some studies[27] but others argue for delta analgesia as well.[26] The differences could be due to different sites with different opioid receptors being accessed in the various studies. The intraventricular administration of kappa opioids in the rat produces analgesia under circumstances where spinal application produces negative effects.

The mechanisms of action of opioids at supraspinal levels is still poorly understood although there are two particular theories which are of interest. One, based on the existence of Diffuse Noxious Inhibitory Controls, holds that the contrast between a discrete pool of activated nociceptive neurones and a surrounding pool of ongoing innocuous activity forms the message perceived by the brain as noxious; supraspinal morphine reduces the contrast rather than the activation of nociceptive neurones so blurring the perception of pain.[28] This would fit well with the idea that lower doses of morphine (which are likely to be acting supraspinally) in man reduce the unpleasant nature of pain without much alteration in the intensity. Spinal opioids would by contrast block the spinal transmission and so reduce both the sensory and affective response. The second theory which is not exclusive of the first, is that cells in the brain stem are turned off by noxious stimuli; this then allows a reflex to occur. Morphine turns on these cells so no reflex results whilst inhibiting a second group of cells which are activated by a noxious stimulus.[29] Both concepts then rely on two distinct effects of morphine on two pools of cells.

The peptidase inhibitors described earlier have actions at supraspinal sites but in this series of studies the effects of the protected enkephalins were likely to be due to actions at the mu receptor.

Opioid mechanisms at a number of other supraspinal sites are likely to be of relevance to analgesic phenomena such as their actions at thalamic levels and the laminar segregation of different receptors in the sensory cortex. The large numbers of opioid receptors in areas such as the solitary tract and adjacent areas are probably related to respiratory effects, cough suppression and nausea and vomiting. Sites in the monoamine nuclei such as the well demonstrated actions of opioids in the locus coeruleus and the ventral tegmental area are likely to be associated with reward processes and so relate to dependence. The relative extent of the unwanted effects caused by selective agonists at the different opioid receptors is of great importance in determining if non-mu opioids will have better spectra of actions as compared to morphine.[23] These studies are difficult since there are few systemically active selective agonists for comparative studies to morphine. However there are good indications that the kappa and delta receptor agonists cause less respiratory depression than mu and that prolonged protection of the enkephalins by the peptidase inhibitors has no dependence liability. This lack of dependence is also seen with kappa agonists but is accompanied by aversive or non-rewarding effects that limit the usefulness of these agents in man.[19] There is no evidence either way at present to determine if these effects of purported kappa opioids are mediated by the kappa receptor or are due to other actions of the drugs since many of the kappa ligands have additional non-opioid effects.

ALTERATIONS IN OPIOID SYSTEMS

The ability of opioids to elicit analgesia in man, to be active on standard tests in animals or effective on acute C fibre or noxious evoked electrophysiological indices (with the exception of certain studies of spinal kappa effects) is not the whole story. It has been clearly established in man that whereas opioids are excellent analgesics in many pain states there are instances where their effectiveness is less than expected. A well established example is the pain from neuropathic origins such as post amputation and nerve injury induced pains where opioids are poorly effective.[30] A paradox is that in animal models where either the pre-synaptic opioid receptors have been removed by prior rhizotomy (electrophysiological)[31] or in a model of postsynaptic activation of nociceptive systems, (behavioural)[32] morphine is still effective, although higher doses than in normal animals are required in the former case. In these situations the antinociceptive effects of morphine are not surprising since there will be not only be the spinal postsynaptic receptors available but also the supraspinal sites. Therefore why are opioids ineffective in similar clinical states? Apart from the problems of animal studies as models for human disorders an explanation for reduced opioid effects may then be not simply the available receptor pool but: (a) release of chemicals such as the non-opioid peptides FLFQPQRFamide or cholecystokinin, known to interfere with opioid actions; or (b) either a loss of inhibitory influences or surfeit of excitatory activity, rendering the opioid controls insufficiently efficacious. If these events did explain the reductions in morphine efficacy they would have to occur at all sites where opioid receptor activation produces analgesia. In the first case the exogenous spinal application of these peptides will prevent mu but not delta mediated neuronal inhibitions,[33] and intrathecal morphine analgesia and as would be predicted, systemic CCK antagonists will enhance systemic morphine analgesia. Thus in situations where there is a release of these peptides one would expect a reduction in morphine effects without requiring any change in opioid receptors number.

In the second situation the use of prolonged nociceptive stimulation has provided some ideas as to the basis for altered opioid function. In inflammatory states there is an increase in the mRNA in the spinal cord for dynorphin and to a lesser extent, for enkephalin with all the cells increasing dynorphin synthesis having a preceding rise in c-fos, a protooncogene.[34] Dynorphin can mimic some of the increases in excitability seen after inflammation, such as the increased nociceptive responses of neurones whilst inhibiting others.[21] In addition the kappa opioid can antagonise the mu receptor in a number of tissues including the spinal cord so potentially contributing to the decreased morphine effectiveness.[35]

The other side of the coin is the increased excitability of cells being hard to counter. There is good evidence that the N-methyl-D-aspartate (NMDA) receptor for the excitatory amino acids can, when activated, induce increased nociceptive responsiveness[36] and so can amplify and extend noxious inputs.[37,38] The enhanced cell responses to noxious stimulation mediated by NMDA mechanisms (the so-called wind-up) are also less sensitive than steady activity to opioids.[10] In inflammatory states where spinal NMDA receptors are operative opioid application is less effective (by about 30%) compared to when given as a pretreatment, where the opioid inhibitions may well prevent the central hyper-responsiveness from being elicited.[39] Interestingly the prior administration of systemic morphine prevents the induction of c-fos produced by noxious inflammatory stimulation.[40] Since the induction of a gene in nociceptive neurones may have far-reaching consequences the pretreatment with opioids may produce benefits outlasting acute analgesia. There is also reduced opioid effectiveness in other central hypersensitive states.[41] The ensemble of these results agree well with clinical findings that in some situations the preventive administration of analgesics including morphine has dramatically better results than when given *post hoc*.[42] The actions of opioids at their various sites may then be useful not only in reducing ongoing nociception but in prevention of untoward neural plasticity since the NMDA receptor may play a critical role in some deleritous maladaptive pain states.[43]

Opioids despite a lack of action at cutaneous sites in undamaged tissue do have actions on the peripheral generation of inflammatory pain suggesting that the consequences of inflammation can induce an additional site of opioid action which is not present in normal tissue. The relative effectiveness of mu, delta and kappa receptor activation to elicit peripheral analgesia varies but in arthritic states all three are active.[44] Thus opioids unable to penetrate the CNS and so being devoid of central side-effects may be good analgesics in inflammatory states via these peripheral sites.

Finally there is now a considerable body of evidence showing that low doses of the opiate antagonist, naloxone can elicit analgesia in a number of animal models whereas higher doses produce hyperalgesia, events that could suggest the existence of presynaptic opioid receptors which control the release of endogenous opioids so that antagonism of this receptor increases opioid levels.[45]

The metabolism of morphine to the 3- and the 6-glucuronides does not signify the end of the analgesia since, although the 3 conjugate is inactive, the morphine-6-glucuronide is considerably more potent than morphine intrathecally in the rat[46] and is also highly effective by the systemic route in man.[47] Thus accumulations of this metabolite will prolong opioid actions even after metabolism of the parent morphine.

The synthesis of non-mu opioids, peptidase inhibitors, opioids with peripheral actions only and adjuncts which would reduce anti-opioid systems will hopefully will lead to alternative therapeutic agents if they can be made in systemically active forms, a goal which is being approached. So from both the viewpoint of therapy and a furthering of our knowledge of nociceptive processes both in the long and short term opioids look likely to remain a subject area of great activity.

REFERENCES

1 Kosterlitz HW. Opioid peptides and their receptors. Proc R Soc 1985; 225: 27–40
2 Kosterlitz HW. Biosynthesis of morphine in the animal kingdom. Nature 1987; 330: 606–607
3 Duggan AW, North RA. Electrophysiology of opioids. Pharmacol Rev 1984; 35: 219–281
4 North RA. Drug receptors and the inhibition of nerve cells. Br J Pharmacol 1989; 98: 13–28
5 McFadzean I. The ionic mechanisms underlying opioid actions. Neuropeptides 1988; 11: 173–180
6 Petrillo P, Tavani A, Verotta D, Robson LE, Kosterlitz HW. Differential postnatal development of μ-, δ- and κ-opioid binding sites in rat brain. Dev Brain Res 1987; 31: 53–58
7 Besson JM, Chaouch A. Peripheral and Spinal Mechanisms of Nociception. Physiol Rev 1987; 67: 67–186
8 Yaksh TL, Nouiehed R. Physiology and Pharmacology of spinal opiates. Ann Rev Pharmacol Toxicol 1985; 25: 433–462
9 Besse D, Lombard MC, Zakac JM, Roques BP, Besson JM. Pre- and postsynaptic distribution of mu, delta and kappa opioid receptors in the superficial layers of the cervical dorsal horn of the rat spinal cord. Brain Res 1990; 521: 15–22
10 Dickenson AH, Sullivan AF. Electrophysiological studies on the effects of the effects of intrathecal morphine on nociceptive neurones in the rat dorsal horn. Pain 1986; 24: 211–222
11 Sullivan AF, Dickenson AH. Electrophysiological studies on the spinal effects of dermorphin, an endogenous μ opioid agonist. Brain Res 1988; 461: 182–185
12 Dickenson AH, Sullivan AF, Knox RJ, Zajac Z, Roques BP. Opioid receptor types in the rat spinal cord: electrophysiological studies with μ and δ opioid receptor agonists in the control of nociception. Brain Res 1987; 413: 649–652
13 Stevens CW, Yaksh TL. Time course characteristics of tolerance development to continuously infused antinociceptive agents in rat spinal cord. J Pharmacol Exp Ther 1989; 251: 216–223
14 McQuay HJ, Sullivan AF, Smallman K, Dickenson AH. Intrathecal opioids, potency and lipophilicity. Pain 1989; 36: 111–115
15 Porreca F, Mosberg HI, Hurst R, Hruby VJ, Burks TF. Roles of mu, delta and kappa opioid receptors in spinal and supraspinal mediation of gastrointestinal transit effects and hot-plate analgesia in the mouse. J Pharmacol Exp Ther 1984; 230: 341–348
16 Schmauss C, Yaksh TL. In vivo studies on spinal opiate receptor systems

mediating antinociception II Pharmacological profiles suggesting a differential association of μ, δ and κ receptors with visceral chemical and cutaneous thermal stimuli in the rat. J Pharmacol Exp Ther 1984; 228: 1–12

17 Sullivan AF, Dickenson AH, Roques BP. δ- opioid mediated inhibitions of acute and prolonged noxious-evoked responses in rat dorsal horn neurones. Br J Pharm 1989; 98: 1039–1049

18 Stevens CW, Weinger MB, Yaksh TL. Intrathecal dynorphins suppress hindlimb electromyographic activity in rats. Eur J Pharmacol 1987; 138: 299–302

19 Millan MJ. k opioid receptors and analgesia. Trends Pharmacol Sci 1990; 11: 70–76

20 Parsons CG, Headley PM. Spinal antinociceptive actions of μ- and κ-opioids; the importance of stimulus intensity in determining 'selectivity' between reflexes to different modalities of noxious stimulus. Br J Pharmacol 1989; 98: 523–532

21 Knox RJ, Dickenson AH. Effects of selective and non-selective κ opioid agonists on cutaneous C fibre evoked responses of rat dorsal horn neurones. Brain Res 1987; 415: 11–19

22 Allerton CA, Smith JAM, Boden PR, Hunter JC, Hill RG, Hughes J. Correlation of ontogeny with function of [3H]U69593 labelled k opioid binding sites in the rat spinal cord. Brain Res 1989; 502: 149–157

23 Roques BP. What are the relevant features of the distribution, selective binding and metabolism of opioid peptides and how can these be applied to drug design? In: Basbaum AI, Besson JM, eds. Towards a new pharmacotherapy of pain. Dahlem Conferenzen. New York: Wiley, 1990 (in press).

24 Dickenson AH, Sullivan AF, Fournie-Zaluski M-C, Roques B. Prevention of degradation of endogenous enkephalins produces inhibition of nociceptive neurones in rat spinal cord. Brain Res 1987; 408: 185–191

25 Yaksh TL, AL-Rodhan NRF, Jenson TS. Sites of action of opiates in production of analgesia. Prog Brain Res 1988; 77: 371–394

26 Heyman JS, Vaught JL, Raffa RB, Porreca F. Can supraspinal δ-opioid receptors mediate antinociception? Trends Pharmacol Sci 1988; 9: 134–138

27 Chaillet P, Coulard A, Zajac JM, Fournie-Zaluski MC, Costentin J, Roques BP. The μ rather than the δ subtype of opioid receptors appears to be involved in enkephalin induced analgesia. Eur J Pharmacol 1984; 101: 83–90

28 Le Bars D, Villanueva L. Electrophysiological evidence for the activation of descending inhibitory controls by nociceptive afferent pathways. Prog Brain Res 1988; 77: 275–300

29 Fields HL, Barbaro NM, Heinricher MM. Brain stem neuronal circuitry underlying the antinociceptive action of opiates. Prog Brain Res 1988; 77: 245–258

30 Arner S, Meyerson BA. Lack of analgesic effect of opioids on neuropathic and idiopathic forms of pain. Pain 1988; 33: 11–23

31 Lombard MC, Besson JM. Attempts to gauge the relative importance of pre- and postsynaptic effects of morphine on the transmission of noxious messages in the dorsal horn of the rat spinal cord. Pain 1989; 37: 335–346

32 Hylden JLK, Wilcox GL. Pharmacological characterization of Substance P induced nociception in mice: modulation by opioid and noradrenergic agonists at the spinal level. J Pharmacol Exp Ther 1983; 226: 398–404

33 Magnuson DSK, Sullivan AF, Simmonet G, Roques BP, Dickenson AH. Differential interactions of cholecystokinin and FLQPQRFamide with μ and δ opioid antinociception in rat spinal cord. Neuropeptides 1990; 16: 213–218

34 Ruda MA, Iadorala MJ, Cohen LV, Young III WS. In situ hybridisation histochemistry and immunocytochemistry reveal an increase in spinal cord dynorphin biosynthesis in a rat model of peripheral inflammation and hyperalgesia. Proc Natl Acad Sci USA 1988; 85: 622–626

35 Dickenson AH, Knox RJ. Antagonism of μ opioid receptor mediated inhibitions

of nociceptive neurones by U50488H and dynorphin 1–13 in the rat dorsal horn. Neurosci Letts 1987; 75: 229–234

36 Evans RH. The pharmacology of segmental transmission in the spinal cord. Prog Neurobiol 1989; 33: 255–279

37 Haley JE, Sullivan AF, Dickenson AH. Evidence for spinal N-methyl-D-aspartate receptor involvement in prolonged chemical nociception in the rat. Brain Res 1990; 518: 218–226

38 Thompson SWN, King AE, Woolf CJ. Activity-dependent changes in rat ventral horn neurons in vitro; summation of prolonged afferent evoked postsynaptic depolarizations produce a D-2-amino-5-phosponovaleric acid sensitive windup. Eur J Neurosci 1990; 2: 638–649

39 Dickenson AH, Sullivan AF. Subcutaneous formalin induced activity of dorsal horn neurones in the rat: differential response to an intrathecal opiate administered pre or post formalin. Pain 1989; 30: 349–360

40 Presley RW, Menetrey D, Levine JD, Basbaum AI. Systemic morphine suppresses noxious stimulus-evoked fos protein-like immunoreactivity in the rat spinal cord. Neuroscience 1991 (in press)

41 Woolf CJ, Wall PD. Morphine sensitive and morphine insensitive actions of C-fibre input on the rat spinal cord. Neurosci Letts 1986; 64: 221–225

42 McQuay H, Dickenson AH. Implications of central nervous system plasticity for pain management. Anaesthesia 1990; 45: 101–102

43 Dickenson AH. A cure for wind-up: NMDA receptor antagonists as potential analgesics. Trends Pharm Sci 1990; 11: 307–309

44 Stein C, Millan MJ, Shippenberg TS, Peter K, Herz A. Peripheral opioid receptors mediating antinociception in inflammation. Evidence for involvement of mu, delta and kappa receptors. J Pharmacol Exp Ther 1989; 248: 1269–1275

45 Kayser V, Benoist JM, Neil A, Gautron M, Guilbaud G. Behavioural and electrophysiological studies on the paradoxical antinociceptive effects of an extremely low dose of naloxone in an animal model of acute and localized inflammation. Exp Brain Res 1988; 73: 402–410

46 Sullivan AF, McQuay HJ, Bailey D, Dickenson AH. The spinal antinociceptive actions of morphine metabolites, morphine-6-glucuronide and normorphine in the rat. Brain Res 1989; 482: 219–224

47 Hand CW, Blunnie WP, Claffey LP, McShane AJ, McQuay HJ, Moore RA. Morphine-6-glucuronide in csf after im and oral administration of morphine: potential analgesic contribution from this metabolite. Lancet 1987; II: 1207–1208

British Medical Bulletin (1991) Vol. 47, No. 3, pp. 703–717
© The British Council 1991

Opioid clinical pharmacology and routes of administration

H J McQuay
Oxford Regional Pain Relief Unit, Abingdon Hospital, Oxford, UK

Opiate prescription is based on titration to effect. This principle is supported by the difference between the laboratory and clinical pharmacologies of opiates. Clinically the presence of nociceptive pain appears to act as a counter to the respiratory depressant effect of opiates, and perhaps the dependence, which are such features in the laboratory.

Factors in choosing between opiates are described; these include onset speed, duration of effect, toxic and active metabolites and specific side-effects. Side-effect comparison between opiates is only satisfactory when the drugs are compared at equianalgesic doses. The kinetic and clinical logic of alternative routes is explored.

Overall there is probably more difference between the effect of the same opiate given by different routes than between the effects of different opiates given by the same route.

Opioids are used primarily to produce pain relief. Although they have been given by every conceivable route, the common ones are oral, intramuscular, intravenous and subcutaneous. The effect of changing route with the same drug may be greater than that of changing drug within the same route.

DIFFERENCES BETWEEN OPIOID LABORATORY AND CLINICAL PHARMACOLOGY

Clinical pain management has emphasized a difference between the clinical and the laboratory pharmacology of opiates. It is as though there is one opiate pharmacology when the opiate is used to counteract pain, and another when it is not.

The respiratory depression which haunts prescribers in acute pain management is seen readily in studies of volunteers who are not in pain. For patients with opiate-sensitive pain, given appropriate doses of opiate, respiratory depression is minimal.[1,2] The balance between pain and opiate respiratory effects is seen clearly in chronic pain. Patients maintained on oral morphine, with no clinical respiratory depression, and who then receive successful nerve blocks, must have their morphine dose reduced. Failure to reduce the dose will result in respiratory depression.[3,4] One explanation is that the respiratory centre receives nociceptive input.[5] Presence of this input counterbalances any respiratory depressant effect of the opiate. Absence of this input, because of the successful nerve block, leaves the respiratory depressant effect of the opiate unopposed.

The clinical message is that opiates need to be titrated against pain. Doses higher than necessary for the relief of pain run the risk of respiratory depression. Prophylactic use of opiates, infusion without regard to pain experienced, doses greater than those required for analgesia (as in deliberate ITU use to facilitate ventilation of a patient), use for purposes other than analgesia (e.g. sedation), or use in non-nociceptive pain, thus all carry potential risk. Concern about respiratory depression should not inhibit the appropriate use of opioids, and that is to provide analgesia when the pain may reasonably be thought to be opiate sensitive. A postoperative patient still complaining of pain when the previous dose can be assumed to have been absorbed needs more drug.

Similarly the drug-seeking behaviour synonymous with street addiction is not found in patients after pain relief with opiates, either in childbirth, or after operations or after myocardial infarction.[6] Street addicts are not in pain. The political message is that medical use of opiates does not create street addicts. Medical use may indirectly increase availability to those who are already addicts, but restricting medical use hurts patients.

UNRESOLVED CLINICAL ISSUES

Unresolved issues[7] in clinical opiate use include the choice of opiate, the decision to prescribe by the clock or as required, tolerance, pain sensitivity to opioids, and choice of route. These are discussed in turn in this section.

Choosing an opiate

Morphine is the standard opiate against which others are judged. Other drugs may act faster, last longer or have a better balance between effect and side-effect for a particular patient. Some of the ways in which opiates differ are shown in Table 1.

Political decisions limit medical availability in many countries. Partial agonists and mixed agonist-antagonists have particular importance in this context because they have lower dependence liability and may be the only permissible agents. Drug availability and prescriber or institution preference may then be major factors in choice.

Efficacy and ceiling effect

The ceiling to analgesic effect is the inability of a drug to relieve pain beyond a certain intensity, despite an increase in dose. This may be due to toxicity at higher doses, to a failure of compliance, or it may be an intrinsic property of the drug.

If increasing the dose increases the incidence of unwanted effects (toxicity) this creates a limit to analgesic efficacy. Codeine and dihydrocodeine are usually classified as 'weak' analgesics occupying an intermediate rung on the analgesic ladder.[8] This weakness is due to unacceptable side effects at the higher doses required to treat severe pain. Pethidine in large doses may produce central nervous system toxicity (*see below*).

Drugs acting as partial rather than pure agonists may be incapable of relieving severe pain. This may be more of a theoretical than a practical bar to use, because the ceiling effect may occur only at high doses. If the dose of drug in each tablet (or ml of solution) is small, and the dose required is large, it may be physically difficult to take or to give the necessary dose.

Speed of onset & duration of action

Fast onset of effect is not a critical factor if the patient is receiving analgesics by-the-clock for chronic pain, but may be relevant for the patient taking the drug when needed for acute or chronic pain. By the intravenous (i.v.) route there is little perceptible difference between onset time for different opiates. Intramuscularly (i.m.), the more lipophilic the drug the faster the onset time.

There is much confusion between kinetics and effect. Short or

Table 1 Properties of some of the opioids used commonly in pain management

Drug	Route	Dose mg	Effect onset min	Duration h	Kinetic $T_{1/2b}$ h	Comments
Morphine	i.m.	10	30–60	3–4	3–5	The standard drug. ↑ M6G, active metabolite, accumulation in renal dysfunction
Heroin	p.o.	60	60–90	3–4		
	i.m.	5–10	80–240	N/A		
	p.o.	50	30–60	3–4		Fast-acting potent drug
Hydromorphone	i.m.	1.5	15–30	4	2–3	
	p.o.	7.5	30–45	4	2–3	
Codeine	i.m.	130	30–60	3–4	N/A	
	p.o.	200	60–90	3–4	N/A	
Oxycodone	i.m.	15	15–30	4		
	p.o.	30	15–30	4		
Levorphanol	p.o.	4	30–60	4–5	12–16	
	i.m.	2	60–90	4–5		
Pethidine	i.m.	75	30–45	3	3–4 (pethidine)	Cirrhosis ↑ bioavailability & ↓ clearance; renal failure ↑ norpethidine, toxic metabolite, accumulation;
	p.o.	300	60–90	4–5	12–16 (norpethidine)	phenytoin ↑ biotransformation; MAO inhibitors excitation, hyperpyrexia & convulsions
Methadone	i.m.	10	30–45	4–5	17–24	Long t1/2b. Rifampicin ↑ biotransformation
Dextromoramide	p.o.	20	20–60	4–5		
Dipipanone	p.o.	10–20	120–240	?		
Pentazocine	p.o.	(5)	45–60	3–4		Psychoto-mimetic effects
	i.m.	60	30–45	3–4	4–5	Cirrhosis ↑ bioavailability and ↓ clearance Low ceiling
Nalbuphine	p.o.	180	30–60	4		
	i.m.	12	30–45	4		
Butorphanol	p.o.	60	30–60	4		Psychoto-mimetic
	i.m.	2	30–45	4	N/A	?ceiling
Buprenorphine	i.m.	0.3	10–20	6–8	3.5	
	s.l.	0.4	30–90	6–8		

long kinetic terminal half-lives are misunderstood as necessarily imputing short or long duration of effect. Claims that fentanyl and cogeners have shorter effect than other i.v. opiates are based primarily on differences in kinetics. Methadone has a long terminal half-life (Table 1). Its effect (given i.v.) may last no longer than that of morphine.[9] This disparity between effect and kinetics may make a safe and effective dose more difficult to find with methadone than morphine, although methods exist.[10] Sustained release oral formulations may prolong the effect duration of opiates, but at the cost of slow onset of effect; morphine slow release tablets give 12 h effect with onset time of 2–4 h, whereas the effect of conventional formulations lasts 4 h and begins at 1 h.

Specific side-effects & metabolism

If an opiate has no specific advantage over morphine and has a specific disadvantage, such as a troublesome side-effect not found with morphine, then there is little logic in choosing that drug in preference to morphine. Any drug which produced fewer side-effects than morphine, at a dose which provided the same degree of analgesia, would be an improvement. High dose fentanyl in cardiac anaesthesia causes less haemodynamic disruption than high dose morphine. For most clinically important side-effects there is no comparative evidence at equivalent analgesic doses to recommend any of the alternatives. Single-dose postoperative studies showed a higher incidence of nausea and vomiting with pethidine,[11] and dysphoria (*see below*) with those mixed agonist-antagonists which have a relatively high affinity for kappa (κ) and sigma (σ) receptors.[12] As with non-steroidal anti-inflammatory drugs, the risk:benefit ratio may be different at equianalgesic dosing within the same patient,[13] but we cannot predict these individual responses.

Dysphoria: Dysphoria occurs with all opiates, but the incidence varies widely between drugs. Pentazocine, butorphanol and nalbuphine have this potential.[14] The greater than 20% incidence with pentazocine and butorphanol contrasts sharply with the 3% incidence seen with other opiates. There is little sense in using an opiate which produces a higher incidence of dysphoria than morphine without any compensating advantage.

Toxic metabolites: Pethidine is metabolised to norpethidine which is toxic.[15] It causes tremor, twitching, agitation and convulsions, and the incidence of these problems increases with multiple dosing and in the presence of impaired renal function.[15,16]

Active metabolite: Whereas diamorphine[17] and morphine-3-glu-curonide (M3G)[18] do not bind to opiate receptors, 6-monoacetyl-morphine, morphine, morphine-6-glucuronide (M6G) and normorphine do. Recent work on the metabolites of morphine has important clinical implications.[19,20] Quantitatively the most important active metabolite is M6G, because M3G and M6G are the major metabolites of morphine in man[21,22] and because of the greater potency of M6G compared with morphine. In rats, M6G is 45 times more potent than morphine intracerebrally and nearly 4 times more potent subcutaneously[23]; intrathecal injection gave potency ratios between 10 and 20.[24] M6G may contribute substantially to the analgesic effect of morphine, in both single and repeated doses.[25-27]

Diamorphine is a classical pro-drug. Without analgesic activity itself, it initiates the 'cascade' into the active 6-monoacetylmorphine, morphine and M6G. Because of the speed of these reactions, there is no clinical advantage over morphine by oral or intramuscular routes, either in terms of greater analgesic efficacy or of improved mood.[17,28] This does not exclude advantage from intravenous, spinal or other routes.

Pathophysiology: Unexpected degree and duration of effect can be obtained with morphine, codeine and dihydrocodeine when they are used in patients with severely impaired renal function.[29] Cumulation of M6G is the probable explanation of this phenomenon. Prolonged respiratory depression has been reported in man in association with negligible plasma concentrations of morphine but with very high concentrations of M3G and M6G.[30] Glucuronidation of morphine is altered little in hepatic failure,[31] but in precoma kinetics[32] and dynamics[33] are altered.

Problems should arise only if a fixed-dose schedule is used without taking account of renal function, or without adequate titration against pain intensity. Drug doses should be decreased markedly if creatinine clearance is less than 30 ml min^{-1}. With less severe renal dysfunction the potential problem emphasizes the need for careful titration, remembering that renal function deteriorates with advancing age. Other pathophysiological problems are shown in Table 1.

Dose equivalence: When changing routes of administration, the dose of the drug must be adjusted, particularly between oral and parenteral routes if the opiate undergoes extensive first pass metabolism. For morphine the effect of a single injected dose was 6 times that of an oral dose.[34] In the multiple dosing context of chronic pain, ratios of 2:1 or 3:1 are used successfully.[35] The active metabolites may contribute more to the analgesic effect with repeated doses than with a single dose.[26,36]

Partial agonists & mixed agonist-antagonists

Partial agonists have less effect via a particular receptor sub-type than a full agonist. Mixed agonist-antagonists combine agonist (full or partial) activity on one or more sub-types with antagonist activity on other(s). Common to the group are lower dependence liability than is found with agonists and a ceiling to their efficacy.

The ability of these drugs to antagonize other opiates has lead to the dogma that they should not be prescribed together with full agonists. The antagonism is however more evident with chronic exposure.[37] Many patients who have been prescribed both full agonist and partial agonist or mixed agonist-antagonist, both at doses within the 'normal' therapeutic range, appear to have additive analgesia.[38] While co-prescription makes little sense because it invites problems unnecessarily, the disparity between the clinical observations and the pharmacological predictions remains to be explained satisfactorily.

The issue of ceiling to efficacy appears to be restrictive only for nalbuphine, for which the ceiling is equivalent to 30 mg morphine. For the other drugs the ceiling is closer to 300 mg morphine equivalence, which is unlikely to be restrictive. Two benefits of efficacy ceiling, on dose-response curves other than analgesia, are that the ceiling for respiratory depression appears to be equivalent to about 20 to 30 mg of morphine, making the drugs theoretically safe in overdosage, and theoretically there should also be a ceiling to constipation.

Prescribe regularly or as required?

Should opiates be given on a fixed 'by the clock' schedule or when the patient asks for them? Given that serious side-effects emerge when the dose is greater than that needed to provide adequate analgesia, the over-riding principle is to titrate to effect. Patient-controlled analgesia shows that this principle is both safe and effective. The principle of titration to effect calls into question the safety of both prophylactic opiate dosing and infusions which take no account of the level of pain intensity.

In acute pain doses have to be given when needed, titrating to effective dose size and interval. In chronic pain when effective dose size and interval are established the doses are given by the clock. Such fixed dose schedules for oral morphine in chronic pain prevent the pain re-emerging. If pain is allowed to re-emerge, the relatively slow onset of analgesic effect of oral morphine means that it takes time to re-establish control.

Tolerance

Tolerance is the need for a bigger dose (or higher plasma concentration) to achieve the same pharmacological effect. The word is often misused in pain management to mean an increase in dose; this is only correct if the pain has not increased. In chronic cancer pain the reason for increasing the dose is usually an increase in the pain.[39] Patients are often maintained satisfactorily on the same oral morphine dosage for months, and this would not be possible if tolerance always occurred.

Genuine tolerance to opiate use does occur in other contexts. Addicts develop tolerance; they, however, use opiates in the absence of pain. Acute tolerance to opiates has been demonstrated in animal studies; control groups given a painful stimulus before the injection of opiate did not develop acute tolerance.[40] The phenomenon of acute tolerance has also been demonstrated in man.[41] Opiate injection before surgery (before the patient is in pain) is common practice, both as premedication and in the anaesthetic room. It does not create clinical problems because any increase in postoperative opiate requirement can be met.

Reports of clinical problems due to tolerance are often hard to interpret. In some cases spinal opiates were used for pain which had failed to respond to opiates given by conventional routes. On the basis of this and other clinical criteria these were opiate insensitive conditions. The second problem with interpretation is in knowing whether the dose being given was the minimum necessary or whether it was more than was needed. If the latter, tolerance would be expected.

The enigma of opiate tolerance reinforces the concept of a dual pharmacology. When the drugs are used in appropriate doses to treat pain which is opiate sensitive, tolerance (like respiratory depression) is not a clinical problem. When opiates are used in the absence of an opiate sensitive pain, or in inappropriately high dosage when the pain is sensitive, then (like respiratory depression) tolerance can occur.

Opiate insensitive pain

In chronic pain not all pains are relieved by opiates.[42,43] A good example is trigeminal neuralgia, in which opiates provide poor pain relief and the anticonvulsant, carbamazepine, works well. Opiate insensitive pain may be defined as pain which does not respond progressively to increasing opiate dose; the commonest causes of opiate insensitive pain are nerve compression and nerve destruction. Studies comparing efficacy of different opiates in chronic pain, or different routes of administration, need to establish the degree of opiate sensitivity of the pain; comparisons in opiate insensitive pain will be meaningless.

Choosing the route

Two clinical issues have become confused in discussion of alternative routes [44]. The first is clinical necessity; some patients may have to be managed by a 'non-standard' route of administration, such as those cancer pain patients who cannot take oral medication. The second is the potential of novel routes to provide better analgesia and/or fewer side-effects than standard routes, so that the novel route supplants the standard. Although the first is clear and logical, the second remains to be proven.

The sublingual and spinal routes are current clinical alternatives to conventional routes of administration. Other proposed routes (nasal, transdermal, inhalational etc.) should be subject to the same questions; what is the kinetic logic of the route, and what is the clinical logic?

Sublingual and buccal opiates

The kinetic logic of the sublingual and buccal routes is that the drug is given without injection but is absorbed systemically (analogous to an intramuscular dose), avoiding any first-pass metabolism, and so increasing relative systemic bio-availability. The real clinical gain is that a given dose should be more predictable both within and between patients than an equivalent oral dose, because it is the variability of first-pass metabolism which makes short-term use of oral opiates difficult. Sublingual buprenorphine provides the best example of the kinetic gain in availability. Postoperatively 0.4 mg sublingually produced analgesia equivalent to 0.3 mg i.m. Relative systemic availability was 55% (range 16 to

94%). The relative systemic availability of oral buprenorphine was about 15%.[45,46]

No kinetic advantage of sublingual use would be predicted for low clearance drugs, and no advantage for sublingual use of methadone, which has a low clearance and high oral availability, was found.[45] Similarly little kinetic advantage was found with sublingual morphine.[45-47] Claims for kinetic advantage with buccal morphine[48] have not been substantiated.[46]

Clinically, sublingual use is an alternative to oral where swallowing is difficult, or to injection when strong opiates are needed in contexts where injection is problematic, such as in children, or in haemophiliacs.

Subcutaneous infusion

Subcutaneous infusions using a battery-driven portable syringe driver[49] are used commonly in terminal care for patients who cannot swallow or have persistent vomiting. Opiates with greater solubility than morphine are used if repeated injections have to be given in cachectic patients.

Spinal opiates

Spinal (generic for intrathecal and extradural) opiate use is contentious, because of the potential for greater morbidity than with conventional routes. Spinal opiates, however, produce pain relief whose quality and duration are greater than that achieved by opiates given by conventional routes. This means that the risk:benefit ratio for spinal opiates must be defined and compared with that for conventional routes.[50] The belief that applying opiate directly into the central nervous system (CNS) produces an absolute difference in analgesia and side-effect incidence compared with conventional routes has little logic behind it; the drugs act on the same receptors however they are given, so that the difference can only be relative. Spinal opiate use has had a strong phenomenological flavour. The appropriate clinical role is unresolved.

Kinetic logic: The kinetic logic of spinal administration is to inject exogenous neurotransmitters close to the CNS to work directly on opiate receptors. Lipophilicity influences the ability to cross the blood-brain barrier;[51] this principle underlies the systemic kinetic differences between drugs, and is circumvented by direct intrathecal application.[52] This is evident in the change in the relative potency of different μ agonists intrathecally compared with i.v. Methadone 10 mg given systemically produces equivalent analgesia to systemic morphine 10 mg. Intrathecally, however, methadone is 18 times less potent than morphine.[52,53] These differences between systemic and spinal dosing have not been applied as they should have been in determining equianalgesic doses.

The benefit of giving opiates extradurally comes from the fraction of the extradural dose which crosses the dura directly. While the kinetics of this fraction will be predictable from intrathecal kinetics, the proportion of drug absorbed systemically will follow the kinetic principles for systemic absorption.[54] For methadone the 'systemic' fraction is equipotent with morphine, but the 'spinal' fraction is not.

The high drug concentrations achieved after lumbar intrathecal injection[55] spread rostrally,[56] and make a combination of spinal and supraspinal effect possible. This may be a necessary combination for adequate analgesia. Systemic absorption from the extradural space would also take the drug to supraspinal receptors. The high csf concentrations, however, also raise the spectre of toxicity. None has been found, either in prolonged monkey studies (4 to 16 months extradural morphine[57]), or in man after 6 months extradural morphine.[58] Use of more potent agents should perhaps be recommended on the basis of fewer non-specific actions until more is known.

Clinical logic: A small dose of morphine given spinally can provide equivalent analgesia to larger doses given orally or by conventional injection routes. The duration of effect of these smaller doses may also be greater. The evidence for opiates other than morphine is confused. The equianalgesic doses of lipophilic opiates given intrathecally are much higher than was realized; 5 mg methadone was not equianalgesic with 0.5 mg morphine,[59] as might be predicted.[52] Similarly with extradural use no clinical advantage was seen with extradural fentanyl compared with i.v.[60,61] These papers emphasize the necessity of systemic controls in extradural studies. Spinal opiates may, however, be more effective in the presence of local anaesthetics.[62]

The major problems encountered in acute pain are itch, urinary retention and respiratory depression. In chronic pain these have not been problematical.[63] Previous opiate exposure seems to minimize the incidence. The claim is made that side-effects may be reduced with spinal use compared with conventional routes, at the

same or greater analgesic effect. Convincing evidence is still necessary, both with drug (morphine) and between drugs. Again, comparison must be made at equianalgesic doses.

Intrathecal or extradural?: The intrathecal route offers certain
availability of the drug in csf when compared with the extradural
route. There is an analogy to the certain availability of the i.v.
route when compared with i.m. Intrathecal administration
requires dural puncture. An extradural catheter might be thought
to have considerable logistic advantage and lower morbidity compared with an intrathecal catheter. There is no comparative
evidence.

REFERENCES

1 Walsh TD, Baxter R, Bowerman K, Leber B. High-dose morphine and respiratory function in chronic cancer pain. Pain 1981; S1: 39
2 Regnard CFB, Badger C. Opioids, sleep and the time of death. Palliat Med
   1987; 1: 107–110
3 Hanks GW, Twycross RG, Lloyd JW. Unexpected complication of successful
   nerve block. Anaesthesia 1981; 36: 37–39
4 McQuay HJ. Potential problems of using both opioids and local anaesthetic
   (letter). Br J Anaesth 1988; 61: 121
5 Arita H, Kogo N, Ichikawa K. Locations of medullary neurons with non-phasic
   discharges excited by stimulation of central and/or peripheral chemoreceptors
   and by activation of nociceptors in cat. Brain Res 1988; 442: 1–10
6 Porter J, Jick H. Addiction rate in patients treated with narcotics. N Engl J
   Med 1980; 302: 123
7 Foley KM. Current Controversies in Opioid Therapy. In: Foley KM, Inturrisi
   CE, eds. Opioid analgesics in Management of Cancer Pain. Advances in Pain
   Research & Therapy, Vol 8. New York: Raven Press, 1986: pp. 3–11
8 Twycross RG, McQuay HJ. Opioids. In: Wall PD, Melzack R, eds. Textbook
   of Pain. Edinburgh: Churchill Livingstone, 1989: pp. 686–701
9 Grochow L, Sheidler V, Grossman S, Green L, Enterline J. Does intravenous
   methadone provide longer lasting analgesia than intravenous morphine? A randomised, double-blind study. Pain 1989; 38: 151–158
10 Sawe J, Hansen J, Ginman C et al. Patient-controlled dose regimen of methadone for chronic cancer pain. Br Med J 1981; 282: 771–773
11 Morrison JD, Hill GB, Dundee JW. Studies of drugs given before anaesthesia
   XV: evaluation of the method of study after 10,000 observations. Br J Anaesth
   1968; 40: 890–900
12 Wallenstein SL, Rogers AG, Kaiko RF, House RW. Nalbuphine clinical analgesic studies. In: Foley KM, Inturrisi CE, eds. Opioid analgesics in the management of cancer pain. Advances in Pain Research and Therapy, Vol. 8. New
   York: Raven Press, 1986: 247–252
13 Kalso E, Vainio A. Morphine and oxycodone hydrochloride in the management
   of cancer pain. Clin Pharmacol Ther 1990; 47: 639–646
14 Houde RW. Discussion. In: Foley KM, Inturrisi CE, eds. Opioid analgesics
   in the management of cancer pain. Advances in Pain Research and Therapy,
   Vol. 8. New York: Raven Press, 1986: 261–263
15 Szeto HH, Inturrisi CE, Houde R, Saal S, Cheigh J, Reidenberg M. Accumulation of norperidine, an active metabolite of meperidine, in patients with renal
   failure or cancer. Ann Int Med 1977; 86: 738–741

16 Boreus LO, Odar-Cederlof I, Bondesson U, Holmberg L, Heyner L. Elimination of meperidine and its metabolites in old patients compared to young patients. In: Foley KM, Inturrisi CE eds. Opioid analgesics in the management of cancer pain, Advances in pain research & therapy, Vol. 8. New York: Raven Press, 1986: pp. 167–169
17 Inturrisi CE, Max M, Umans J et al. The pharmacokinetics of heroin in patients with chronic pain. N Engl J Med 1984; 310: 1213–1217
18 Christensen CB, Jorgenson LN. Morphine-6-glucuronide has high affinity for the opioid receptor. Pharmacol Toxicol 1987; 60: 75–76
19 Osborne R, Joel S, Trew D, Slevin M. Morphine and metabolite behavior after different routes of morphine administration: demonstration of the importance of the active metabolite morphine-6-glucuronide. Clin Pharmacol Ther 1990; 47: 12–19
20 McQuay HJ, Carroll D, Faura CC, Gavaghan DJ, Hand CW, Moore RA. Oral morphine in cancer pain: influences on morphine and metabolite concentrations. Clin Pharmacol Ther 1990; 48: 236–244
21 Boerner U, Abbott S, Roe RL. The metabolism of morphine and heroin in man. Drug Metab Rev 1975; 4: 39–73
22 Sawe J, Dahlstrom B, Paalzow L, Rane A. Morphine Kinetics in Cancer Patients. Clin Pharmacol Ther 1981; 30: 629–635
23 Shimomura K, Kamata O, Ueki S et al. Analgesic effect of morphine glucuronides. Tohoku J Exp Med 1971; 105: 45–52
24 Sullivan AF, McQuay HJ, Bailey D, Dickenson AH. The spinal antinociceptive actions of morphine metabolites morphine-6-glucuronide and normorphine in the rat. Brain Res 1989; 482: 219–224
25 Hand CW, Blunnie WP, Claffey LP, McShane AJ, McQuay HJ, Moore RA. Potential analgesic contribution from morphine-6-glucuronide in csf. Lancet 1987; ii: 1207–1208
26 McQuay HJ, Moore RA, Hand CW, Sear JW. Potency of oral morphine. Lancet 1987; ii: 1458–1459
27 Osborne R, Joel S, Trew D, Slevin M. Analgesic activity of morphine-6-glucuronide. Lancet 1988; i: 828
28 Twycross RG, Wald SJ. Longterm use of diamorphine in advanced cancer. In: Bonica JJ, Albe-Fessard D, eds. Advances in pain research and therapy, Vol. 1. New York: Raven Press, 1976: pp. 653–661
29 McQuay HJ, Moore RA. Be aware of renal function when prescribing morphine. Lancet 1984; ii: 284–285
30 Osborne RJ, Joel SP, Slevin ML. Morphine intoxication in renal failure: the role of morphine-6-glucuronide. Br Med J 1986; 292: 1548–1549
31 Patwardhan RV, Johnson RF, Hoyumpa A, Sheehan JJ, Desmond PV, Wilkinson GR, Branch RA et al. Normal metabolism of morphine in cirrhosis. Gastroenterology 1981; 81: 1006–1011
32 Hasselstrom J, Eriksson S, Persson A, Rane A, Svensson JO, Sawe J. The metabolism and bioavailability of morphine in patients with severe liver cirrhosis. Br J Clin Pharmacol 1990; 29: 289–297
33 Laidlow J, Read AE, Sherlock S. Morphine tolerance in hepatic cirrhosis. Gastroenterology 1961; 40: 389–396
34 Houde RW, Wallenstein SL, Beaver WT. Clinical measurement of pain. In: G De Stevens. Analgesics. New York and London: Academic Press; 1965: pp. 75–122
35 Twycross RG, Lack S. Symptom control in far advanced cancer; Pain relief. London: Pitman; 1983
36 Hanks GW, Aherne GE, Hoskin PJ, Turner P. Explanation for potency of repeated oral doses of morphine. Lancet 1987; 2: 723–725
37 Houde RW, Wallenstein SL, Rogers A. Interactions of pentazocine and morphine. (Analgesic Studies Program of the Sloan-Kettering Institute for Cancer

Research). In: Report of the 34th Annual Scientific Meeting of the Committee on Problems of Drug Dependence. New York: National Academy of Science, 1972: pp. 153–164

38 Levine JD, Gordon NC. Synergism between the analgesic actions of morphine and pentazocine. Pain 1988; 33: 369–372

39 Kanner RM, Foley KM. Patterns of narcotic drug use in cancer pain clinic. Ann N Y Acad Sci 1981; 362: 162–172

40 Colpaert FC, Niemegeers CJE, Janssen PAJ, Maroli AN. The effects of prior fentanyl administration and of pain on fentanyl analgesia: tolerance to and enhancement of narcotic analgesia. J Pharmacol Exp Ther 1980; 213: 418–426

41 McQuay HJ, Bullingham RES, Moore RA. Acute opiate tolerance in man. Life Sci 1981; 28: 2513–2517

42 McQuay HJ. Pharmacological treatment of neuralgic and neuropathic pain. Cancer Surv 1988; 7: 141–159

43 Arner S, Meyerson BA. Lack of analgesic effect of opioids on neuropathic and idiopathic forms of pain. Pain 1988; 33: 11—23

44 McQuay HJ. The logic of alternative routes. J Pain Symptom Manag 1990; 5: 75–77

45 McQuay HJ, Moore RA, Bullingham RES. Sublingual morphine, heroin, methadone and buprenorphine: kinetics and effects. In: Foley KM, Inturrisi CE, eds. Opioid analgesics in the Management of Cancer Pain. Advances in Pain Research & Therapy, Vol. 8. New York: Raven Press. 1986: pp. 407–411

46 Weinberg DS, Inturrisi CE, Reidenberg B et al. Sublingual absorption of selected opioid analgesics. Clin Pharmacol Ther 1988; 44: 335–342

47 Pannuti F, Rossi AP, Iafelice G. Control of chronic pain in very advanced cancer patients with morphine hydrochloride administered by oral, rectal, and sublingual route. Pharmacol Res Commun 1982; 14: 369–380

48 Bell MDD, Murray GR, Mishra P, Calvey TN, Weldon BD, Williams NE. Buccal morphine—a new route for analgesia. Lancet 1985; i: 71–73

49 Oliver DJ. The use of the syringe driver in terminal care. Br J Clin Pharmacol 1985; 20: 515–516

50 Anonymous. Spinal opiates revisited. Lancet 1986; i: 655–656

51 Herz A, Teschemacher HJ. Activities and sites of antinociceptive action of morphine like analgesics. Adv Drug Res 1971; 6: 79–119

52 McQuay HJ, Sullivan AF, Smallwood K, Dickenson AH. Intrathecal opioids, potency and lipophilicity. Pain 1989; 36: 111–115

53 Dickenson AH, Sullivan AF, McQuay HJ. Intrathecal etorphine, fentanyl and buprenorphine on spinal nociceptive neurones in the rat. Pain 1990; 42: 227–234

54 Bullingham RES, McQuay HJ, Moore RA. Intrathecal and extradural narcotics. In: Atkinson RS, Langton Hewer C, eds. Recent Advances in Anaesthesia and Analgesia 14. Edinburgh: Churchill Livingstone; 1982: 141–156

55 Moore RA, Bullingham RES, McQuay HJ, Allen MC, Cole A. Spinal fluid kinetics of morphine and heroin. Clin Pharmacol Ther 1984; 35: 40–45

56 Moulin DE, Inturrisi CE, Foley KM. Epidural and intrathecal opioids: cerebrospinal fluid and plasma pharmacokinetics in cancer pain patients. In: Foley KM, Inturrisi CE, eds. Opioid analgesics in the management of cancer pain. Advances in Pain Research and Therapy, Vol. 8. New York: Raven Press; 1986: pp. 369–383

57 Yaksh TL. Spinal opiate analgesia; Characteristics and principles of action. Pain 1981; 11: 293–346

58 Meier FA, Coombs DW, Saunders RL, Pageau MG. Pathologic anatomy of constant morphine infusion by intraspinal silastic catheter. Anesthesiology 1982; 57: 206

59 Jacobson L, Chabal C, Brody MC, Ward RJ. Intrathecal methadone 5 mg and

morphine 0.5 mg for postoperative analgesia: a comparison of the efficacy, duration and side effects. Anesth Analgesia 1989; 68: S132

60 Loper KA, Ready BL, Downey M et al. Epidural and intravenous fentanyl infusions are clinically equivalent after knee surgery. Anesthes Analgesia 1990; 70: 72–75

61 Ellis DJ, Millar WL, Reisner LS. A randomised double-blind comparison of epidural versus intravenous fentanyl infusion for analgesia after cesarian section. Anesthesiology 1990; 72: 981–986

62 Akerman A, Arwestrom E, Post C. Local anaesthetics potentiate spinal morphine antinociception. Anaesthesia 1988; 67: 943–948

63 Coombs DW. Management of chronic pain by epidural and intrathecal opioids: newer drugs and delivery systems. In: Sjostrand UH, Rawal N, eds. Opioids in Anesthesiology and Pain Management. International Anesthesiology Clinics, Vol. 24, 1986: pp. 59–74

British Medical Bulletin (1991) Vol. 47, No. 3, pp. 718–731
© The British Council 1991

Opioid-responsive and opioid-non-responsive pain in cancer

G W Hanks*

Department of Palliative Medicine, United Medical and Dental Schools of Guy's and St Thomas's Hospitals, St Thomas's Hospital, London, UK

Cancer pain in general responds in a predictable way to analgesic drugs and drug therapy is the mainstay of treatment, successfully controlling pain in 70–90% of patients. The two major problem areas are pain associated with nerve damage, and 'incident' (movement-related) bone pain. Nerve damage pain tends not to respond well to morphine or other opioids. The difficulty with severe incident pain is that if the dose of opioid is titrated sufficiently to relieve the pain on weight-bearing or on movement and is then given regularly at this level, it is too much for the patient at rest. The patient may then experience excessive side-effects at rest, but still have pain on movement. Other examples of pain which may be resistant to treatment with opioid analgesics are bladder and rectal tenesmus, pancreatic pain, and pain associated with decubitus ulcers or other superficial ulcers subjected to pressure or shearing forces. Management of non-opioid-responsive pain may include a variety of treatments involving adjuvant analgesic drugs and non-drug measures.

Most pain in cancer can be controlled using orally-administered analgesics and adjuvant drugs. It is reported that 70–90% of patients with cancer pain respond to pharmacological manage-ment[1-3] and this response may be sustained for months or years.[4] Such high response rates are not universally achieved and the main

---

*Sainsbury Professor of Palliative Medicine.

reasons for failure are inexperience and lack of knowledge of the simple principles of effective analgesic use (now being widely disseminated by the WHO[5]). It is relevant to keep this in mind in any discussion of so-called opioid-responsive and non-responsive pain. A proportion of apparently unresponsive pains merely require more effective use of the available drugs.

That said, there are a hard core of patients whose pain is not well controlled with opioid analgesics. The term opioid-non-responsive pain has been coined in recent years to describe this phenomenon. The term is not altogether satisfactory because it is too categorical, implying that a pain either **does** respond to opioid analgesics or **does not**. Rarely is there such a clear distinction in clinical practice with the latter group.

Another complication is that a pain may respond to opioid analgesics but may not be well managed by using the drugs in a conventional manner. 'Incident' (movement related) bone pain is the main example of this type of problem: if the dose of opioid is titrated sufficiently to control pain on movement and then given regularly at this level, it is too much for the patient at rest and will cause excessive side-effects.

Opioid-responsive and opioid-non-responsive pain are often equated with nociceptive and non-nociceptive pain, and in general this seems to be a valid rule of thumb as the basis for the differentiation.[6] Nociceptive pain responds to anti-nociceptive measures, which in pharmacological terms means analgesics. Non-nociceptive pain does not respond in a straightforward manner to analgesic drugs. Some hold that this is an absolute lack of response,[7] whilst others suggest that it is relative, and that if a sufficient dose of opioid is used at least a partial response will be obtained. This controversy is academic because clinically one is usually dealing with a mixed picture and this means that invariably an opioid analgesic will be part of the therapeutic regimen.

The clinical definition of opioid non-responsive pain embraces rather more than whether or not a pain is **sensitive** to opioid analgesics. It implies also a differential response in an individual, in which the patient does not derive adequate analgesia, but does experience other pharmacological actions of the opioid drug (as unwanted effects). Much rarer is the patient who does not experience any pharmacodynamic effect at appropriate therapeutic doses. Usually the balance between analgesia and unwanted effects produced by regular oral morphine weighs very much towards analgesia. Unwanted effects are in general easily managed without exceptional measures and are not dose-limiting.

Thus the distinction between opioid-responsive and opioid-non-responsive pain in cancer cannot be couched in precise terms. It encompasses the concept of **sensitivity** to treatment with opioid analgesics, but also implicit is the balance between analgesia and unwanted effects. A working definition is that opioid non-responsive pain is pain which is inadequately relieved by opioid analgesics given in a dose which causes intolerable side-effects despite routine measures to control them.

OPIOID-RESPONSIVE PAIN: CURRENT MANAGEMENT

Morphine is the strong opioid analgesic of choice used according to well-proven principles. It is given by mouth, the dose is tailored to the individual patient, doses are repeated so that the pain is prevented from returning, and there is no arbitrary upper limit.

Dose-titration

Morphine is available in three formulations for oral use: an elixir, a tablet (only recently introduced in the United Kingdom) and a controlled release tablet. (The first two are sometimes referred to as 'immediate or normal release' to distinguish them from the latter.)

An immediate-release formulation is preferable for dose titration. Peak plasma concentrations are achieved within the first hour with the elixir[8] but are slightly delayed with the standard tablet.[9] Both formulations give a rapid effect with a duration of about 4 hours. In contrast controlled release morphine tablets produce delayed peak plasma concentrations at 2–4 hours after administration, the peak is attenuated,[8] and the duration of effect is 12 hours. This means that with this preparation it is difficult both to assess the adequacy of analgesia in order to adjust the dose during the dose-finding period, and to make rapid dose changes.

Dose range

We have used doses of morphine elixir ranging from 2.5 mg 4-hourly to 2000 mg 4-hourly (and are aware of anecdotal reports of much higher doses). This range of almost a thousand-fold to achieve the same endpoint is remarkable and not seen in any other area of therapeutics.

Dose must be adjusted against effect, either until control of pain is achieved or side-effects become intolerable. The majority of patients will require 200 mg per day or less,[10–12] and very few will need high doses, but there is no definable maximum.

There is thus considerable inter-individual variation in the response to oral morphine. Some of the factors which contribute to this[13,14] are the severity of the pain, the type of pain, the affective components of pain, previous analgesic use, age and pharmacokinetic parameters. However, no complicated dose formula is necessary in order to determine the right dose for an individual patient. By titrating the dose against effect all of these factors will be taken into account. The simplest method of dose titration is to prescribe a four-hourly dose (based on previous analgesic use) and at the same time allow top-up doses of the same size for 'breakthrough' pain as frequently as necessary. After 24 or 48 hours the daily requirements may be reassessed and the regular 4-hourly dose adjusted as necessary.

Maintenance

Once a patient's morphine dose requirements have been determined, maintenance treatment will usually be with a controlled release tablet formulation. Most experience has been with a tablet designed for twice daily administration (MST Continus, MS Contin)[15] though others are now becoming available.

Patients with progressive disease and increasing pain may require continual adjustment of dose. For many patients, however, there is a period of stability during which dose requirements are unchanged or need only small adjustments.[4,16] Pharmacological tolerance appears to be rare, for reasons which we do not really understand. There are ample data to show that many patients may go for several months or sometimes years with little change in their morphine dosage.

Adverse effects

Constipation is an almost invariable adverse effect of morphine but should never be a reason for discontinuing the drug. It should be anticipated and treated prophylactically with adequate laxatives. Occasional patients do not become constipated.

Nausea and vomiting occurs in a half to two-thirds of patients taking oral morphine[17] but is variable in intensity and usually easy to control if it does develop. In many patients it is an initiation side-effect and may resolve with continued use of morphine. A small proportion of patients get severe nausea and vomiting which seems to be caused either by gastric stasis or increased vestibular sensitivity,[18] and which may occasionally prove intractable to treatment with conventional antiemetic drugs.

Sedation is frequent at the start of treatment but in the majority of patients resolves within a few days. Hallucinations and confusion are relatively unusual but may occur particularly in elderly patients, and once developed tend to persist unless the dose is reduced or the drug discontinued. This is the most likely adverse effect to necessitate a change in drug or route, though severe sedation or severe nausea and vomiting may also prompt such a move.

Our approach with intractable adverse effects is to change to an alternative strong opioid agonist, and we use phenazocine. This drug is methadone-related, has a longer duration of action of 6–8 hours, but is less flexible in dosage because it is only available as a 5 mg tablet (equivalent to 25 mg oral morphine). Often a change to phenazocine allows pain control to be achieved without the previously troublesome adverse effects associated with morphine.

If adverse effects persist we would move to spinal administration, preferably with intrathecal morphine. This is rare and has been necessary in less than 1% of our 450 admissions a year.

Adverse effects with oral morphine are more likely in the absence of pain. We have suggested that pain acts as a physiological antagonist of the CNS depressant effects of opioid analgesics[10] and that clinically this can be demonstrated in relation to respiratory depression.[19] McQuay has proposed that a possible explanation for this is that the respiratory centre in the medulla receives nociceptive input.[20,21] However, clinical experience suggests that this rule does not apply only to respiratory depression. It appears that a balance is usually achieved between nociceptive pain and the adverse effects of opioid analgesics, so that analgesia is achieved without intolerable unwanted symptoms. In the absence of such pain, adverse effects can become a major problem and such a development should prompt a re-evaluation of the patient.

This thesis is based on anecdotal clinical experience and requires more careful systematic documentation but if it is right it can explain a number of clinical observations.

Therapeutic failure with oral opioids

Non-opioid responsive pain will normally be defined by the development of intolerable adverse effects associated with inadequate analgesia. In this circumstance it is reasonable to ask three questions: 'If the opioid is administered by another route will efficacy (i.e. opioid-sensitivity) be improved?'; 'If the opioid is administered by another route will adverse effects be less?'; and 'Will an alternative oral opioid be either more effective or produce less side-effects?'

The subject of different routes of administration is discussed in detail elsewhere in this issue (*see* McQuay) but opinions remain divided. Most controversy surrounds the use of spinal administration and whether or not efficacy is enhanced by this route. There is no dispute that analgesia may be obtained with spinal opioids using much smaller doses, and that it has a longer duration, and (in the case particularly of intrathecal administration) is associated with a lesser incidence of systemic adverse effects. Some also suggest that the quality of analgesia is improved but a recent extensive review of published data suggests that, 'There is no conclusive evidence that opioids injected extradurally or intrathecally provide analgesia superior to that produced with other routes of administration.'[22]

Our approach is to use spinal administration of opioids in the management of a patient who has a demonstrably opioid-sensitive pain, but who develops intolerable side-effects with systemic administration of morphine or an alternative drug such as phenazocine.

There is no good evidence that efficacy is dependent on route of administration: in general, morphine has equal efficacy if given in appropriate dosage by oral, parenteral or spinal routes. There are always exceptions which prove the rule and there are certainly differences in dose requirements, speed of onset of action, duration of analgesia, and adverse effects which are dependent on the route of administration. However, if pain appears to be unresponsive to morphine by mouth, it is unlikely that changing the route will produce a response, unless there are obvious problems with absorption by the oral route in particular patients.

Alternatives to oral morphine

As indicated above we use phenazocine as our first alternative to oral morphine in patients unable to tolerate the latter drug. We do not have quantitative data to present at this time to support this practice but our anecdotal experience is that frequently this manoeuvre works in achieving analgesia without disabling side-effects.

From time to time controversy has arisen over whether one opioid is more effective than another. There has for example in recent years been a long-running debate in several countries (particularly Canada and Australia) as to whether or not diamorphine is more effective than morphine. The evidence suggests that when relative potency is taken into account (i.e. using 'equianalgesic' doses) there is no difference in efficacy either between these two drugs, or between morphine and other strong opioids.

Opioid-irrelevant pain

In some patients the complaint of pain is more a reflection of social, psychological, or spiritual turmoil rather than a result of physical injury or damage. Such pain is not best treated with morphine and has been characterized as 'opioid-irrelevant pain' (by Hinton, quoted by Kearney[23]). Such pain may present as opioid-non-responsive pain. It may dominate a particular individual, or more commonly may form a component of many patients' complaint of pain. It needs always to be kept in mind.

OPIOID NON-RESPONSIVE PAIN

The two most difficult areas in cancer pain management are nerve damage pain and incident bone pain.[24] There are other cancer pain syndromes which respond poorly or not at all to opioid analgesics. These include bladder and rectal tenesmus, perineal pain associated with pelvic malignancy, pancreatic pain, and pain associated with decubitus ulcers or other superficial ulcers subjected to pressure or shearing forces.

Nerve damage pain

Nerves may be damaged by infiltration or compression by tumour, or as a result of viral infection, or by treatment with surgery, radiotherapy or chemotherapy. The resulting pain is often extremely difficult to treat.

The terminology here is confusing: neuralgia, neuropathic pain, neurogenic pain and deafferentation pain are all terms which are used interchangeably but may mean different things to different people. Neurogenic pain is discussed in detail elsewhere in this issue (*see* McMahon, Charlton, Devor, Wall, Bowsher) but several points are worthy of emphasis here.

Neuropathic pain appears to be relatively insensitive to opioids,[6] though as discussed above this is probably not an absolute phenomenon. Peripheral nerve lesions are often associated both with neuropathic pain and nerve trunk pain[25] which **is** likely to be responsive to opioids. Thus nerve damage is invariably associated with both nociceptive and non-nociceptive pain, and it is important that opioid analgesics are not automatically eschewed when a diagnosis of nerve pain is made. The usual step-wise approach and dose-titration of opioid should be employed, but at the same time alternative treatments may be required.

Nerve damage pain may include a sympathetic component and sympathetic blocks may be helpful.[26] In the management of the other components of neuropathic pain treatments should be targeted at specific symptoms:[27] hyperaesthesia and allodynia (pain due to a non-noxious stimulus); lancinating dysaesthesiae; and burning, crawling or compressing sensations. A variety of drug[28] and non-drug treatments[29] may need to be tried.

Corticosteroids are frequently not considered, yet may produce substantial improvement in neuropathic symptoms in cancer patients. Corticosteroids inhibit the production of prostaglandins and also by blocking the action of lipo-oxygenase, of leukotrienes. The reduction of inflammation, inflammatory oedema and hyperaemia surrounding a tumour mass may relieve the pressure on a nerve, or within a nerve bundle where there is infiltration by tumour. Corticosteroids may also reduce the abnormal sensitivity of nociceptive nerve endings resulting from inflammatory processes associated with a tumour or metastasis, and they have also been shown to reduce neuroma hyperexcitability.[30] Whatever the mechanism, useful palliation of symptoms is often achieved. An adequate dose of steroid is necessary in order to be sure not to miss a treatment effect (dexamethasone 4 mg bd or more).

On the basis of a similar rationale nonsteroidal antiinflammatory drugs may produce at least a partial response,[31] though corticosteroids are more predictable. If corticosteroids do alleviate symptoms and the mechanism is thought likely to be relief of nerve compression (for example radicular pain associated with vertebral metastases) treatment with radiotherapy should also be considered since a longer-lasting effect may be obtained without steroid-related side-effects.

Psychotropic and anticonvulsant drugs, and other 'membrane-stabilizers' are discussed elsewhere. An important point to make here is that polypharmacy and iatrogenic problems are major deterrants to the use of these drugs in this patient population. Patients with nerve pain begin with the balance between unwanted drug effects and analgesia from conventional analgesics leaning towards unwanted effects. The addition of non-conventional analgesics with potent side-effect-producing potential may make a barely manageable situation quite impossible. These factors must be carefully weighed, and the application of antidepressants and anticonvulsants should perhaps be a little more cautious than is usual at present. Doses should start low and, as with morphine, there may be wide inter-individual variation in the therapeutic level which will be required. Thus the dose may need to be titrated through a considerable range for some patients.

The most recent addition to the armamentarium of membrane-stabilizers is the anti-arrythmic flecainide.[32] Our experience has been that a small number of patients with pain refractory to all other treatments have obtained substantial benefit from this drug. Caution and careful screening of patients is necessary because of its potential cardiotoxicity but the activity of flecainide in these particularly difficult pain states holds promise for future developments with this group of drugs.

Incident pain

Incident pain is a term most commonly applied to pain on weight-bearing or movement, but may also be caused by swallowing, micturition, defaecation, cough or some other action of the patient.[33] Frequently such 'breakthrough' pains can be adequately coped with by the use of a top-up dose of opioid, and invariably patients should have this made available to them. Our practice is to use the usual 4-hourly dose or equivalent, repeated as frequently as the breakthrough pain necessitates. It seems illogical to use a smaller dose though all sorts of formulae have been advocated.[33] There are no pharmacokinetic data to support one particular practice but our rationale is that the breakthrough dose should be **adequate** to relieve the breakthrough pain, and adverse effects are not a problem when our approach is adopted.

Much more difficult to manage is severe bone pain on movement caused by skeletal metastases. The usual approach to management of radiotherapy[34] and morphine plus a non-steroidal antiinflammatory drug,[35] perhaps supplemented with a diphosphonate, will control most bone pain at rest. The dose of morphine should be titrated up to allow as much mobility as possible, but if the dose goes too high the patient is likely to experience excessive adverse effects at rest when there are no pain-provoking factors in play. This situation is not easily dealt with by using breakthrough doses of morphine because the movement-related pain is likely to be repetitive but unpredictable.

Alternative strategies are necessary. Orthopaedic intervention by pinning of long bones, spinal stabilization, or even joint replacement may be justified in order to enable an otherwise bed-bound patient to mobilize.[36] Obviously the prognosis and the general condition of the patient have to be carefully weighed but the benefits may be considerable. In patients for whom surgical intervention is not possible, external stabilization using splints or orthoses may be sufficient to allow mobilization without excruciating pain.

This is an area where the physiotherapy and occupational therapy members of the team have much to offer. The correct use of mobility aids, careful analysis and instruction of ergonomic principles, and adaptations of the patient's home environment are all likely to be more productive than continual pharmacological manipulation. These are difficult problems, sometimes inadequately managed in spite of all of the efforts of the multidisciplinary team. It is an important area for future research.

Pancreatic pain

The incidence of carcinoma of the pancreas has doubled in the UK in the last 40 years (and trebled in the USA) and is now the third most common site of cancer in the gastro-intestinal tract in men. Pain is common, occurring in up to 90% of patients at some stage, often at presentation.

Pain associated with carcinoma of the pancreas can frequently be problematical and occasionally appears to be quite unresponsive to opioid analgesics. Coeliac plexus block is often advocated for such pain[37,38] and indeed has been described as 'the best known and widely accepted nerve block for pain'.[3]

Two recent reviews draw somewhat different conclusions about the utility of this procedure. The first reports retrospectively on extensive experience over a 4-year period in 101 patients: good pain relief was obtained in 80% of the patients with malignant disease (not all had carcinoma of the pancreas).[39]

However, a review of the literature on coeliac plexus block published over the last 25 years points out that the duration of analgesia, long-term morbidity and relative analgesic efficacy of coeliac plexus block are difficult to definitively categorise from the published papers and the authors question its usefulness.[40] However they also point out that in experienced hands it is a safe procedure.

There are certainly substantial data similar to that cited in the first review above, claiming high response rates with this technique. Our experience is that there are widely differing responses to this procedure in different patients. However, significant benefit is frequently obtained at the risk of minimal morbidity, and this is the crucial equation. We would continue to use this block in patients with upper abdominal pain of whatever aetiology that is not well controlled using oral opioids. There is a need for more rigorous evaluation of the technique and comparison with other methods of treatment. Some have suggested, for example, that epidural morphine may be more effective for pancreatic pain (Husebo, personal communication). This remains an open question.

Other opioid non-responsive pains

It is not uncommon to have a patient receiving large doses of opioid analgesics who still complains of severe discomfort from pressure sores. To some extent pressure sore pain is incident pain because it is most troublesome when the patient is lying on the affected area, or brushing against it. Drugs are not the mainstay of treatment. There is substantial literature on this subject and it is not appropriate to go into detail here. Prevention is the main concern[41] but once developed, pressure sores will require the use of special mattresses or beds and careful wound management. The usual approach to analgesia is to use a combination of an opioid with a non-steroidal antiinflammatory drug, but this is probably the least important measure in relieving pain caused by pressure sores.

Bladder and rectal tenesmus, and occasionally a proctalgia fugax-like severe episodic rectal spasm may complicate pelvic tumours and these spasmodic pains tend not to respond well to opioid analgesics, partly because of their intermittent nature. A variety of pharmacological treatments are available and are usually tried with increasing desperation, but often to no avail. Simple solutions should be sought first. With bladder tenesmoid pains it is important to rule out infection or direct irritation by catheter, tumour, debris or blood clot. If none of these are present our approach to drugs would be to try first a non-steroidal antiinflammatory, and as second-line a smooth muscle relaxant such as flavoxate, dicyclomine or propantheline. Sedative phenothiazines, anxiolytic drugs and antidepressants have been advocated but we have not found them particularly helpful.

A recent paper reports impressive results in a small series of patients who underwent bilateral chemical lumbar sympathectomy for rectal tenesmoid pain.[42] About 80% (10 out of 12) of the patients achieved complete relief of pain. This is a safe technique associated with low morbidity and should certainly be kept in mind when faced with a patient with this difficult pain complaint.

Other pharmacological remedies have been advocated for non-malignant rectal spasm,[43] but this is another area which needs more research. It is important to recognize that current drug treatments may be ineffectual, and to avoid subjecting patients to endless changes in their drugs. A joint approach to management is required involving not just a consideration of pharmacological and nerve blocking measures but input from the whole multidisciplinary team. An alert, mobile patient with normal bowel function and taking a good diet is less likely to have intractable pain than if he were drowsy, bed-bound, constipated and miserable. Nursing, physiotherapy, occupational therapy and dietitian colleagues may all have an important role in the management of rectal spasm. Nerve blocks are covered in the last chapter (Wells & Miles) of this issue.

CONCLUSION

Most pain in cancer should be easily relieved because it responds in a predictable way to opioid analgesic drugs. Pain which does not respond so well can usually be at least ameliorated by the judicious use of adjuvant analgesics, non-drug measures, and the active involvement of the multidisciplinary team.

REFERENCES

1 Takeda F. Results of field-testing in Japan of the WHO draft interim guidelines on relief of cancer pain. Pain Clinic 1986; 1: 83–89

2 Ventafridda V, Tamburini M, Caraceni A, De Conno F, Naldi F. A validation study of the WHO method for cancer pain relief. Cancer 1987; 59: 851–56

3 Wells JCD. The use of nerve destruction for relief of pain in cancer: a review. Palliat Med 1989; 3: 239–247

4 Walker VA, Hoskin PJ, Hanks GW, White ID. Evaluation of WHO analgesic guidelines for cancer pain in a hospital-based palliative care unit. J Pain Symptom Manag 1988; 3: 145–49

5 World Health Organization. Cancer pain relief. Geneva: World Health Organisation, 1986

6 Arner S, Meyerson BA. Lack of analgesic effects of opioids on neuropathic and idiopathic forms of pain. Pain 1988; 33: 11–23

7 Twycross RG. Opioid analgesics in cancer pain: current practice and controversies. Cancer Surv 1988; 7: 29–53

8 Poulain P, Hoskin PJ, Hanks GW et al. Relative bioavailability of controlled release morphine tablets (MST Continus) in cancer patients. Br J Anaesth 1988; 61: 569–574

9 Sawe J, Dahlstrom B, Rane A. Steady-state kinetics and analgesic effect of oral morphine in cancer patients. Eur J Clin Pharmacol 1983; 24: 537–542

10 Hanks GW, Twycross RG. Pain, the physiological antagonist of opioid analgesics. Lancet 1984; i: 1477–8

11 Twycross RG, Lack SA. Symptom Control in Far Advanced Cancer: Pain Relief. London: Pitman, 1983

12 Walsh TD. Oral methadone for relief of chronic pain from cancer. N Engl J Med 1982; 306: 990

13 Hanks GW, Hoskin PJ. Opioid analgesics in the management of pain in patients with cancer. A review. Palliat Med 1987; 1: 1–25

14 Hoskin PJ, Hanks GW. Morphine: pharmacokinetics and clinical practice. Br J Cancer 1990; 62: 705–707

15 Hanks GW. Controlled-release morphine (MST Contin) in advanced cancer: the European experience. Cancer 1989; 623: 2378–2382

16 Twycross RG. Clinical experience with diamorphine in advanced malignant disease. Int J Clin Pharmacol 1974; 9: 184–198

17 Hanks GW. Antiemetics for terminal cancer patients. Lancet 1982; ii: 1410

18 Gutner LB, Gould WJ, Batterman RC. The effects of potent analgesics upon vestibular function. J Clin Invest 1952; 31: 259–266

19 Hanks GW, Twycross RG, Lloyd JW. Unexpected complication of successful nerve block. Anaesthesia 1981; 36: 37–39

20 McQuay HJ. Potential problems of using both opioids and local anaesthetic. Br J Anaesth 1988; 61: 121

21 Arita H, Kogo N, Ichikawa K. Locations of medullary neurons with non-phasic discharges excited by stimulation of central and/or peripheral chemoreceptors and by activation of nociceptors in cat. Brain Res 1988; 442: 1–10

22 Morgan M. The rational use of intrathecal and extradural opioids. Br J Anaesth 1989; 63: 165–188

23 Kearney MK. Experience in a hospice with patients suffering cancer pain. In: Doyle D, ed. Opioids in the treatment of cancer pain. Royal Society of Medicine Services International Congress and Symposium Series No. 146. London: Royal Society of Medicine Services Limited, 1990: pp. 69–74

24 Hanks GW (Editor). Pain and cancer. Cancer Surv 1988; 7: 1–222

25 Asbury AK, Fields HL. Pain due to peripheral nerve damage: a hypothesis. Neurology 1984; 34: 1587–1590

26 Churcher MD. Cancer and sympathetic dependent pain. Palliat Med 1990; 4: 113–116

27 Hanks GW, Lloyd JW. Postherpetic neuralgia. In: Hopkins A, ed. Major Problems in Neurology: Headache—problems in management. London: Saunders, 1988: pp. 164–191

28 McQuay HJ. Pharmacological treatment of neuralgic and neuropathic pain. Cancer Surv 1988; 7: 141–159
29 Filshie J. The non-drug treatment of neuralgic and neuropathic pain of malignancy. Cancer Surv 1988; 7: 161–193
30 Devor M, Govrin-Lippmann R, Raber R. Corticosteroids reduce neuroma hyperexcitability. In Fields AL, Dubner R, Cervero F, eds. Advances in pain research and therapy Vol 9. New York: Raven Press, 1985: pp. 451–455
31 Vecht Ch J. Nociceptive nerve pain and neuropathic pain. Pain 1989; 39: 243–244
32 Dunlop R, Davies RJ, Hickley J, Turner P. Analgesic effects of flecainide. Lancet 1988; i: 420–421
33 Portenoy RK, Hagen NA. Breakthrough pain: definition, prevalence and characteristics. Pain 1990; 41: 273–281
34 Hoskin PJ. Scientific and clinical aspects of radiotherapy in the relief of bone pain. Cancer Surv 1988; 7: 69–86
35 Hanks GW. The pharmacological treatment of bone pain. Cancer Surv 1988; 7: 87–101
36 Galasko CSB. The role of the orthopaedic surgeon in the treatment of bone pain. Cancer Surv 1988; 7: 103–125
37 Lebovitz AH, Lefkowitz M. Pain management of pancreatic carcinoma: a review. Pain 1989; 36: 1–11
38 Filshie J, Golding S, Robbie DS, Husband JE. Unilateral computerized tomography guided celiac plexus block: a technique for pain relief. Anaesthesia 1983; 38: 498–503
39 Hanna M, Peat SJ, Woodham MJ, Latham J, Gouliaris A, Di Vadi P. The use of coeliac plexus blockade in patients with chronic pain. Palliat Med 1989; 4: 11–16
40 Sharfman WH, Walsh TD. Has the analgesic efficacy of neurolytic celiac plexus block been demonstrated in pancreatic cancer pain? Pain 1990; 41: 267–271
41 Young JB. Aids to prevent pressure sores. Br Med J 1990; 300: 1002–1004
42 Bristow A, Foster JMG. Lumbar sympathectomy in the management of rectal tenesmoid pain. Ann R Coll Surg Engl 1988; 70: 38–39
43 Boquet J, Moore N, Lhuintre JP, Boismare F. Diltiazem for proctalgia fugax. Lancet 1986; i: 1493

British Medical Bulletin (1991) Vol. 47, No. 3, pp. 732–742
© The British Council 1991

Pain: Psychological and psychiatric factors

C J Main
Salford Behavioural Medicine Research Unit & Rheumatic Diseases Centre,
University of Manchester, Manchester, UK

C C Spanswick
Salford Behavioural Medicine Research Unit & Pain Relief Centre,
Hope Hospital, Salford, UK

Recent research in the field of chronic pain has highlighted
the importance of the assessment of psychological factors
as part of the overall assessment of the chronic pain
patient. Reliance only on self report of pain is inadequate.
A number of different approaches have been taken to
psychological evaluation, ranging from formal assessment
of psychiatric illness to self-report questionnaires and
clinical evaluation. In this chapter, each of the major types
of assessment is described and illustrated with examples of
specific tests or assessment instruments.

The chapter highlights research which has attempted to
appraise the relative value of different sorts of
psychological information in assessment of the impact of
pain or in the patient's response to treatment.
Recommendations for the design of a simple
comprehensive system for chronic pain are made.

During the last decade the role of psychological factors in the
genesis and maintenance of pain problems has been increasingly
recognized. It has become increasingly evident that the medical
model does not explain the varying levels of disability in patients
with the same level of objective damage in chronic illness. While
in cancer pain patients the level of self report of pain seems to be
related to the amount of ongoing tissue damage, in patients with
chronic benign pain this is quite clearly not the case. It would
seem, therefore, that other factors must play an important part in
the presentation of a patient with chronic benign pain.

Persistent pain and limitation in activities of daily living, as with any other life stress, will eventually have a psychological impact on the patient. Once the pain and disability has progressed beyond the acute phase, the chronic pain patient may become progressively more demoralized and distressed.[1] The effects of repeated investigations and failed treatment magnify the distress still further and may lead to magnified illness presentation in the form of inappropriate responses to physical examination or inappropriate symptomatology.[2] In addition to distress, anger and inappropriate illness behaviour, confusion and misunderstanding may arise. Patients do not realize that much treatment is purely empirical and do not understand why others with apparently similar symptoms may be offered quite different investigations or treatment. Due to this complex background, psychological management and treatment (of whatever nature) must be based on an adequate assessment of the patient, made with an acknowledgement of the special needs of the chronic pain patient.[3]

Chronic pain does not seem to bear a one-to-one relationship to underlying sensory or physiological dysfunction. Unfortunately, most approaches to treatment still seem to be based on this assumption. Chapman[4] provided an interesting four-dimensional model of human pain which incorporated noxious sensory input, a motivational–emotional dimension, the conceptual appraisal associated with the noxious input, and the socio-cultural dimension within which the pain patient understands and communicates his pain. Thus the nature of chronic pain is being considered from an increasingly broad perspective and assessment has reflected this trend.

PERSONALITY FACTORS

Most of the early studies into psychological factors have involved an investigation of personality structure. The most frequently used test has been the M.M.P.I., devised originally for the identification of psychiatric abnormality (or the probability of psychiatric 'caseness'). The M.M.P.I. has been used in three main ways:

1. *Diagnostically* to differentiate patients with or without organic findings considered adequate to explain the extent of their reported pain;
2. *Descriptively* to describe the psychological features of pain patients; and
3. *Predictively* to assess outcome of various sorts of treatment.

A number of studies have demonstrated poor discriminative validity of the test in terms of 'functional' versus 'organic' and indeed it has been recommended that the terms 'functional', 'organic' and 'mixed' should no longer be used.[5]

Early descriptive studies reported on the frequency of elevations particularly on the first three clinical scales (Hypochondriasis:Hs, Depression:D, and Hysteria:Hy), sometimes referred to as the 'neurotic triad'. The most common descriptive configuration has been the 'Conversion-V' typified by clear elevations on the Hs and Hy scales with a lesser elevation on D. The clinical interpretation and validity of the scales, however, has been seriously questioned.[6] More specifically, Fordyce[7] described an 'illusion of homogeneity' in the M.M.P.I. profiles of low back patients. Elevations on scales Hs, D and Hy are found relatively consistently in pain patients, but the high misclassification indicates that its use (if at all) should be confined to comparisons of groups of patients rather than be used as a basis for decision making with individual patients. Naliboff et al.[8] concluded that '*The data do not support attempts at ... a low back pain or chronic pain personality profile apart from the emotional disturbance associated with chronic limitation and disruption of activity*'. The scales seem to reflect impact of disease rather than psychological status.

The Eysenck Personality Questionnaire or E.P.Q.[9] is the latest in a series of British personality tests. It has been used in the UK in studies of cancer pain. However, a recent study[10] has shown that long-term personality traits as assessed by the E.P.Q. are much less strongly associated with patients level of disability than are measures of distress or magnified illness behaviour (*see below*).

A more specific questionnaire is the Illness Behaviour Questionnaire or I.B.Q.[11] The latest version consists of 62 items giving scores on 7 different scales of which the best known are perhaps General Hypochondriasis and Disease Conviction. The scales have been used widely in studies of pain patients and in general discriminate pain patients from normals, but a recent study[12] has highlighted major statistical problems in the construction of the scales.

It would appear that the initial promise of the investigation of general personality factors in pain has not been fulfilled.[10]

PSYCHIATRIC FACTORS

It is common for patients with chronic illness to be classified as hysterical, hypochondriacal, or mentally ill, particularly if they display, what is considered by the physician, to be exaggerated behaviour or if no obvious demonstrable 'organic' cause for their symptoms can be found. Such patients are frequently referred to psychiatrists in desperation. Most general psychiatrists will return the patient stating that they are not mentally ill and that many of their problems will improve when the pain is cured. The Mental Illness Model does not explain the problem of chronic pain and classifying patients as neurotic, hysterical or hypochondriacal helps neither the patient nor the doctor in their management.

While it is common for patients with chronic pain to use depressive language and even present with some depressive symptomatology this does not mean that they are psychiatrically depressed. The distress shown by chronic pain patients often contains depressive features but Ward[13] has made a clear distinction between clinical depression and pain. Tyrer[14] reports a survey from the Mayo Clinic which showed that although 53% of patients were depressed on admission to the pain centre only 2% were depressed on discharge and he (Tyrer) concludes that the role of the psychiatrist in the Pain Clinic is in fact limited as such patients often improve with no specific pharmacological or other treatment for their depression. Patients do, however, respond to a multidisciplinary pain programme based more on a 'learned-helplessness' model.

Psychodynamic models of pain are characterized by variants of the concept of conversion hysteria, in which a physical symptom is given a psychological interpretation. Thus, for example, the diagnosis of psychogenic low back pain assumes a primary psychological aetiology for the pain. It is assumed that the patient is unable to face an unresolved psychological conflict, and that the back pain is a symptom of this. Chronic pain has been described as the 'somatic expression of unresolved psychic pain' and as a variant of a depressive mood disorder. A number of other early psychoanalytic formulations of the nature of back pain are reviewed by Turk and Flor.[15] Much of the early theorising would now be considered fanciful and lacking a scientific basis.

It could be argued that almost any therapeutic interaction can be described in psychodynamic, cognitive or behavioural terms but the essence of the psychodynamic approach is the central importance given to the therapist-patient relationship in treatment. Tunks and Merskey[16] provide a clear account of the role of psychotherapy in the treatment of pain. They distinguish primarily between supportive and dynamic psychotherapy, although they also review the role of family therapy and group therapy.

Supportive psychotherapy is a feature of good medicine, and it could be argued that it represents a component in any successful rehabilitation programme. Although perhaps an essential component in a good doctor-patient relationship, and certainly helpful in the building of confidence and alleviation of distress, it would not normally be considered powerful enough as a technique in its own right to make much impact on pain, coping skills or physical functioning.

The role of dynamic insight-oriented therapy is much less well established and is not considered to be the most appropriate treatment for the majority of chronic pain sufferers[16] although success has been claimed for psychotherapy in conjunction with other pain treatment modalities.

Studies of psychiatric patients have shown a high level of reported pain. Understandably this led to attempts to construe pain as an aspect of psychiatric illness and attempts to establish the clinical basis for the psychogenic pain syndrome. Differences between psychiatric patients who report pain and chronic pain patients who are distressed were not fully appreciated. Fordyce[17] has drawn attention to the importance of the distinction between pain behaviour and suffering. Many patients are willing to acknowledge distress as well as pain, and may welcome treatment directed at the alleviation of distress, but the clinical and psychological history of most back pain patients, for example, make a primary psychogenic diagnosis implausible. In the alleviation of distress and suffering, several different psychological therapies may be employed, but psychotherapy seems to offer no unique advantage as far as back pain is concerned. Insight-oriented approaches to therapy are not favoured by most patients and there is no evidence for their specific efficacy in the treatment of back pain.

PSYCHOLOGICAL DISTRESS

It is frequently observed that patients with chronic pain report a wide variety of symptoms, although these are not necessarily accompanied by the direct acknowledgment of emotional difficulties. Main[18] produced a test of heightened autonomic or somatic awareness, or 'somatic anxiety'. The precise clinical interpretation of heightened somatic awareness is not entirely clear, since there is not a close relationship with subjective anxiety, but the test was constructed on the basis only of symptoms which differentiated chronic back pain patients from normals. In a recent study,[10] it was shown that this test in conjunction with a measure of depressive symptomatology[19,20] was highly associated with patients' level of disability. It has been suggested that increased attention to bodily mechanisms may be a fundamental cognitive mechanism underlying illness behaviour. Certainly, it is associated with depressive symptomatology, and magnified illness presentation[2] and with poor response to surgery.[21] Heightened somatic awareness has usually been understood as a form of distress.

Depressive symptoms are associated with chronic stress of any sort and are certainly a well-recognized concomitant of chronic pain.[1] The incidence of depressive symptoms is widely variable, and dependant not only on the population studied, but on the diagnostic and descriptive criteria used. A distinction is generally made, however, between endogenous depression and non-endogenous or reactive depression. Only a minority of chronic pain patients (2–14% in various studies) are thought to be endogenously depressed, but approximately 25% of chronic patients seem to have significant depressive symptoms. The depressive symptoms do not seem, however, to constitute a classic reactive depression, as commonly understood by the mental illness model, as discussed above. With chronic pain patients, treatment by psychotropic antidepressant medication appears to be ineffective and responses to treatment are not related to improvement of depression.[13] Depressive symptoms are associated with chronicity and the amount of failed treatment[22] and are associated with 'catastrophising'.[23] Research at present in progress suggests that it may be possible to identify certain clusters or types of patients on the basis of these fairly simple scales. It appears that it may be possible to identify at an early stage patients likely to develop chronic illness.

PSYCHO-PHYSIOLOGICAL ASSESSMENT

In chronic pain patients, general physiological hyperactivity is associated with changes in autonomic nervous activity. Flor et al.[24] have suggested that some chronic pain may result from the interaction of personally relevant stressful events and an underlying physiological predisposition to respond to stress with heightened muscle tension in particular groups of muscles. They found that back pain patients, in contrast with non-back pain patients and healthy controls, displayed elevations and delayed return to baseline only in their paravertebral musculature and only when discussing personally relevant stresses. Flor and Turk[25] have suggested that there is an identifiable subset of patients with chronically elevated stress-related paraspinal EMGs and a slow return to baseline levels.

There is a clear need to clarify the precise nature and role of psychophysiological variables in the development, maintenance and response to treatment in chronic pain. Recent advances in computer technology make this a realistic possibility.

ILLNESS BEHAVIOUR

Psychological investigations have also included investigations of various aspects of pain behaviour. The general principles of Learning Theory were found to be applicable to human behaviour and behavioural analysis of problems of chronic pain and invalidism has led to treatment programmes designed to replace inappropriate behaviour patterns with more adaptive (and appropriate) responses to chronic pain and disease. The general approach is well described elsewhere.[7]

There are both experimental and clinical approaches to the assessment of illness behaviour in low-back pain. Keefe and his colleagues[26] have developed an observational method incorporating a 10-minute standardized sequence of movements which are video-taped and rated according to a set of pain behaviour categories (such as grimacing, and guarding) by trained observers. This method is now being used in the studies of low-back pain and of rheumatoid arthritis. There are a number of behavioural checklists currently available, but these tend to be much too heterogeneous for routine clinical application.

In low-back pain a set of inappropriate responses to physical examination have been identified and integrated into a systematic assessment of the patient. The inappropriate signs test, in conjunction with an assessment of inappropriate symptomatology provide an overall assessment of magnified illness presentation or inappropriate illness behaviour which can be carried out during a routine examination of the low-back pain patient. In general these signs and symptoms are vague, ill-localized and lack the expected relationships with time, physical activity and anatomy. They are best interpreted as signs of distress. These are often misinterpreted as signs of malingering.[20]

It has been shown that the effect of distress and inappropriate illness behaviour increases with duration of symptomatology and with the number of specialists seen. Levels of inappropriate symptomatology are a function of the amount of previous unsuccessful conservative treatment.[22] Distress and illness behaviour also have been identified in the outcome of surgery for low-back pain[21] and in patients' use of narcotics.

BELIEFS ABOUT PAIN AND PAIN CONTROL

The concept of 'locus of control' has been widely influential in the study of the relationship between expectations and behaviour. The original 23 item questionnaire was used to give individuals a score on the I–E dimension, with high scorers (internals) expecting reinforcement to come from their own behaviour and low scorers (externals) expecting reinforcement to come from external forces outwith their control.

Health locus[27] has been shown to be predictive of response to psychological therapy, such as biofeedback, for TMJ pain and headache, and in relaxation training for hypertension.

In general it would appear that 'internals' show lower levels of symptomatology (both physical and psychological) and respond better to treatment than 'externals', but the magnitude of the relationship is unclear and research studies suggest that the influence of health locus may be stronger in relationship to compliance with health education and lifestyle-change programmes than to response to disease or outcome of treatment, when it may be affected by specific features of the health care context rather than by more general beliefs about health.

The Modified Health Locus of Control Questionnaire (MHLC) has been adapted (Crisson and Keefe[28]) for use with pain patients by substituting 'pain' for 'health' in the questionnaire. In the latter study of chronic pain patients, patients who regarded treatment outcome to be determined by chance rated their abilities to control and decrease pain as poor. They also exhibited greater psychological distress and were more likely to report depression, anxiety and obsessive–compulsive symptoms. Furthermore, their results indicated a significant relationship between locus of control and the specific cognitive coping strategies used by the patient.

Recently, a new Pain Locus of Control Questionnaire (PLC)

has been produced.[29] The scales are sensitive to change on Pain Management Programmes and are predictive of future consulting behaviour.

COGNITIVE COPING STRATEGIES

Chronic pain is a stressor and how people cope with stress depends in part on how they appraise the situation. As far as chronic pain is concerned, eliminating the source of stress (i.e. pain) may not be possible, but in order to cope better with it, the person may have to modify his appraisal.[30,31] It has been shown that specific thoughts are associated with lower pain tolerance and cognitive distortions are related (independent of disease severity) to depression and levels of disability, both in chronic low back pain patients and in rheumatoid arthritics. Cognitive therapy is designed to help patients identify and correct distorted conceptualisations; and is often incorporated into cognitive-behavioural therapy.[32]

Recently particular attention has been directed at cognitive coping strategies. They can be broadly grouped into the use of imagery techniques, self-statements (as in stress–inoculation training) and attention–diversion techniques. It has been suggested that patients may require a variety of coping strategies. The most widely used assessment at present is the Coping Strategies Questionnaire or CSQ.[22] Poor coping strategies have been associated with increased levels of functional impairment, pain, depression, state anxiety[22,33] and response to psychological treatment.[33] Patients who were externally controlled scored more highly on the 'Helplessness' scale, reported less effective coping strategies in controlling or decreasing pain levels, were likely to catastrophize and avoid increasing their activity to cope with pain.

CONCLUSIONS

In the assessment of chronic patients and the planning of their treatment, far too much emphasis is placed on the self-report of pain. This is often the only measurement of outcome. There is, therefore, a need for adequate multidimensional assessment of pain patients both prior to treatment and in the evaluation of outcome. Specifically it is important to distinguish psycho-social factors from physical factors. This is essential in the planning of treatment. A large number of psychological tests are available, but not all have been adequately constructed and validated on the chronic pain patient population.

Skilled and sensitive handling of patients with chronic problems is essential. Physical procedures which fail to provide the promised effect are not innocuous but may produce a significant traumatising effect and therefore should not be offered in isolation from any other treatment unless there is clear evidence that they will be helpful. There is a need to move away from the standard disease model towards an illness model in which the role of distress and coping abilities are given at least equal importance to the physical disease characteristics.

RECOMMENDATIONS

1. It is necessary to consider physical, psychological and socio-economic factors in the assessment of chronic pain patients.

2. Physical assessment should incorporate standardised procedures based on careful physical examination, a detailed clinical history (including the patient's response to previous treatment), present level of disability and current drug usage.

3. Psychological assessment should include an evaluation of the patient's level of distress, beliefs about pain and treatment, and magnified illness behaviour.

REFERENCES

1 Sternbach RA. Pain patients: traits and treatment. New York: Academic Press, 1974
2 Waddell G, Main CJ, Morris EW et al. Chronic low back pain, psychological distress and illness behaviour. Spine 1984; 9: 209–213
3 Loeser JD, Seres JL, Newman RI. Interdisciplinary, multimodal management of chronic pain. In: Bonica JJ, ed. The management of pain, 2nd edn. Philadelphia: Lea and Febinger, 1990
4 Chapman RC. Psychological aspect of pain patient treatment. Arch Surg 1977; 112: 767–772
5 Bradley LA, Prieto EJ, Hopson L et al. Comment on 'Personality organisation as an aspect of back pain in a medical setting'. J Person Assess 1978; 42: 573–578
6 Watson D. Neurotic tendencies among chronic pain patients: an MMPI item analysis. Pain 1982; 14: 365–385
7 Fordyce WE. Behavioral Methods for Chronic Pain and Illness. St. Louis: CV Mosby, 1976
8 Naliboff BD, Cohen MJ, Yellen AN. Does the MMPI differentiate chronic illness from chronic pain? Pain 1982; 13: 333–341
9 Eysenck HJ, Eysenck SBG. Manual of the Eysenck Personality Questionnaire. Sevenoaks, Kent: Hodder & Stoughton, 1975

10 Main CJ, Waddell G. Personality assessment in the management of low back pain. Clin Rehab 1987; 1: 139–142

11 Pilowsky I, Spence ND. Patterns of illness behaviour in patients with intractable pain. J Psychosom Res 1975; 19: 279–287

12 Main CJ, Waddell G. Psychometric construction and validity of the Pilowsky Illness Behaviour Questionnaire, Pain 1987; 28: 13–25

13 Ward NG. Pain and depression In: Bonica JJ, ed. The management of pain. 2nd edn. Philadelphia: Lea and Febinger, 1990

14 Tyrer S. The role of the psychiatrist in the pain clinic. Bull R Coll Psych 1985; 9: 135–156

15 Turk DC, Flor H. Etiological theories and treatments for chronic back pain. II Psychological models and interventions. Pain 1984; 19: 209–233

16 Tunks ER, Merskey H. Psychotherapy in the management of chronic pain. In: Bonica JJ, ed. The management of pain. 2nd edn. Philadelphia: Lea and Febinger, 1990

17 Fordyce WE. Learned pain: pain as behaviour. In: Bonica JJ, ed. The management of pain. 2nd edn. Philadelphia: Lea and Febinger, 1990

18 Main CJ. The Modified Somatic Perception Questionnaire. J Psychosom Res 1983; 27: 503–514

19 Zung WWK. The Self-Rating Depression Scale. Arch Gen Psych 1965; 12: 63–70

20 Waddell G. Understanding the patient with back pain. In: Jayson MIV, ed. The lumbar spine and back pain. 3rd edn. Edinburgh: Churchill Livingstone, 1987

21 Waddell G, Morris EW, DiPaola M, et al. A concept of illness tested as an improved basis for surgical decisions in low back disorders. Spine 1986; 11: 712–719

22 Waddell G, Bircher M, Finlayson D, et al. Symptoms and signs: physical disease or illness behaviour? Br Med J 1984; 289: 739–741

23 Rosenstiel AK, Keefe FJ. The use of coping strategies in chronic low back pain patients: relationship to patient characteristics and current adjustments. Pain 1983; 17: 33–44

24 Flor H, Turk DC, Birbaumer N. Assessment of stress-related psychophysiological responses in chronic back pain patients. J Consult Clin Psychol 1985; 53: 354–364

25 Flor H, Turk DC. Psychophysiology of chronic pain: do chronic pain patients exhibit symptom-specific psychophysiological responses? Psych Bull 1989; 105: 215–259

26 Keefe FJ. Block AR. Development of an observation method for assessing pain behaviour in chronic low back pain patients. Behav Ther 1982; 13: 363–375

27 Wallston KA, Wallston BS, DeVellis R. Development of the multidimensional health locus of control (MHLC) scales, Hlth Educ Monog 1978; 6: 160–170

28 Crisson JE, Keefe FJ. The relationship of locus of control to pain coping strategies and psychological distress in chronic pain patients. Pain 1988; 35: 147–154

29 Main CJ, Wood PLR, Spanswick CC. et al. The Pain Locus of Control Questionnaire. (Submitted)

30 Beck AT, Rush AJ, Shaw BR, et al. Cognitive therapy of depression. New York: Guildford Press, 1979

31 Turk DC, Meichenbaum D, Genest M. Pain and behavioural medicine: a cognitive-behavioural perspective, New York: Guilford Press, 1983

32 Turner JA, Romano JM. Cognitive-behavioral therapy. In: Bonica JJ, ed. The management of pain. 2nd edn. Philadelphia: Lea & Febinger, 1990

33 Turner JA, Clancy S. Strategies for coping with chronic low back pain: relationships to pain and disability. Pain 1986; 24: 355–364

British Medical Bulletin (1991) Vol. 47, No. 3, pp. 743–761
© The British Council 1991

Psychological approaches in chronic pain management

C E Pither M K Nicholas
St. Thomas' Pain Management Centre, St. Thomas' Hospital, London, UK

Psychological factors are contributory to the genesis and maintenance of many chronic pain syndromes. Treatment can be delivered either as one component of multimodal therapy or as the sole approach in a pain management programme. This distinction is important as it has a bearing on the goals of treatment, which in the latter situation is to improve management of the pain and encourage the patient to take more responsibility for their treatment, rather than cure the illness.

Treatment typically comprises elements of operant conditioning, where activity and performance can be substantially improved, and cognitive therapy where the thoughts and emotions associated with the pain are tackled, leading to diminution of distress. Relaxation training is also of benefit.

The documented success of these techniques in various settings suggests that psychological treatment should be considered a necessary component of any multidisciplinary clinic offering therapies to chronic pain sufferers.

PSYCHOLOGICAL APPROACHES IN CHRONIC PAIN MANAGEMENT

The last chapter has detailed compelling evidence for the contribution of psychological factors to many chronic pain syndromes. It is apparent therefore that appropriate treatment will include psychological elements. Many practitioners in this country, schooled in the rigid medical model of illness[1] and unfamiliar with the work of health psychologists, tend to view the identification of psychological factors as an indication for a psychiatric referral. While some such patients may have a DSM III[2] psychiatric diagnosis[3] and be best served by conventional psychiatric treatment, this is not the case for the majority. Many patients with chronic pain have difficulty accepting treatment in a psychiatric setting for understandable reasons: they may not feel believed, they may feel rejected by 'real' doctors and they may not be able to accept the implication of an 'emotional' disorder. In addition, conventional psychiatric treatments (such as the use of antidepressants, anxiolytics and psychotherapy) have not been found to be broadly successful in chronic pain. For these reasons this chapter will not discuss further the treatment of chronic pain in a traditional psychiatric setting, but will concentrate on the more widely used psychological techniques relevant to the resources of a multidisciplinary pain clinic. (For a fuller discussion of the psychiatric treatment of chronic pain see Merskey[4]) The actual form of the treatment will, of course, depend upon both the results of the assessment outlined in the previous chapter, and the available resources. The chapter will begin by considering the settings in which psychological treatments are applied—as they largely determine the type of treatment employed and, possibly, their effectiveness. This section will be followed by a brief outline of the main psychological treatments and a discussion of the ways in which they can be delivered. Finally, the effectiveness of psychological treatments will be considered and recommendations for their use in clinical settings will be made.

Psychological treatments are typically employed in two main ways: either as one among many treatments a patient may be receiving, or as the sole treatment once other approaches have been ruled out. The former may be called a 'mixed model' and the latter a 'single model'. In deciding on which approach to employ, the practitioner should consider a number of issues.

Mixed model

For example, typical multidisciplinary pain clinic, where psychological treatments are given simultaneously with other modalities, such as medication, nerve blocks, acupuncture, etc.

In this model the treatment is aimed at diminishing the neurophysiological or nociceptive aspects of the pain with traditional medical approaches (such as nerve blocks, TENS etc.), while concommitant psychological interventions aim at dealing with the psychological issues identified on initial assessment. These may include attempts at changing unhelpful behaviours, trying to improve inappropriate thought patterns, and general supportive therapy. One advantage of this model is that it incorporates manoeuvres aimed at diminishing the pain *per se*. The nature of the medical input, however, implicitly risks maintaining the patient in a semi, if not totally passive role. This may ultimately limit the success of the psychological treatment, which is attempting to encourage greater self-reliance. Thus, the two aspects (the medical and psychological) of this approach could well be in conflict, to the possible detriment of the patient. Clearly, such multidisciplinary approaches need to be well co-ordinated and the purpose of each aspect of treatment carefully explained to the patient.

Single model

For example, pain management programmes, in which psychological considerations provide the guiding principles of the treatment.

In particular, this model attempts to share the responsibility for the treatment with the patient, making them an active participant in the treatment package. The practitioner is no longer seen as the potential provider of a cure, but as an educator and resource provider from whom the patient obtains the skills to make the necessary behavioural, cognitive and emotional changes necessary to improve their management of their pain. Such a model is the basis for most pain management programmes. It should be stressed that the aim of this approach is not to cure the illness, but to help the patient function optimally despite the persisting pain. The aims of pain management are listed in Table 1.

The distinction between these two models has an important bearing on the nature and possible outcomes of psychological treatments. Most medical specialists in the pain field, overly familiar with the passive but demanding patient, do not find it easy to deny pleas for further treatment. This may, however, be necessary. Approaches aimed at returning the responsibility for the management of their illness to the patient cannot be tried in the same way as acupuncture or TENS, as one of a list of possible treatments, which can be passed over if not successful. With every such trial the clinician is essentially reinforcing the view that

Table 1 Goals of a pain management programme

1. Increase the range and level of daily activities including reducing time spent resting and lying down
2. Increase physical fitness in terms of:
   power
   endurance
   flexibility
3. Improve management of pain by patient by e.g.:
   reduce tendency to overdo things by improved pacing
   learn and utilise a relaxation technique
4. Increase confidence in ability to function and cope
5. Eliminate unhelpful cognitions concerning pain. Challenge such thoughts with more realistic thinking
6. Reduce level of pain behaviours
7. Reduce or eliminate powerful analgesics, antidepressants and transquilisers
8. Improve understanding of chronic pain and relevant medical conditions
9. Improve sleep and eliminate inappropriate sedatives
10. Eliminate unnecessary aids such as corsets, collars and crutches
11. Return to work if appropriate
12. Reduce long term health care utilization

improvement is primarily the responsibility of the clinician and that the patient has little contribution to make. Attempting further blocks or procedures, (or renewing the search for a cure), can at a stroke undermine the best efforts of the most well organized psychological treatments which are aimed at enhancing self-sufficiency.

This is particularly important for follow up visits when a patient may be having a setback, claim the pain 'is much worse than ever before', and plead for further treatment. The skills required to handle this situation, with appropriate advice, the suggestion of relevant management techniques, and reinforcement of the patients achievements, need to be aquired by physicians treating chronic pain patients who have received psychological treatment.[5]

TREATMENT TECHNIQUES

A range of psychological treatment techniques have been employed with chronic pain patients. In practice, most clinicians will use a mixture of different techniques with a given patient, depending on the results of both the initial and ongoing assessments of the case. Despite their differences all psychological interventions involve a reconceptualisation of the pain and associated problems.[6] This is an essential element if the patient is to accept the approach and to make sense of the treatment. While the actual content will vary according to the approach being used, most boil down to investigating how psychological factors are contributing to the problem and how the therapist can help the patient to deal with them. The following section will describe only the most widely studied treatments reported in the literature.

Operant–behavioural

This approach is derived from research on learning and emphasizes learning by doing and the use of response-contingent reward or reinforcement to encourage specified behaviours. The first formal applications of the operant approach were described by Fordyce and his colleagues.[7,8] In operant programmes patients set specific activities and exercises as goals which are achieved in a step-like fashion. All steps towards these goals are reinforced by the treatment staff with praise and attention. Eventually, providing the goals are meaningful to the patient, their achievement will also reinforce the patient's efforts, though family and friends may also agree to assist in this regard. At the same time, pain behaviours (e.g. lying down for excessive periods during the day, complaining about pain, etc.) do not receive undue attention lest they be encouraged. The goals of each patient are reviewed regularly by the staff, together with the patient, and raised (or lowered) in terms of frequency or amount depending on progress. For example, with an exercise routine, the patient starts at a level they can manage comfortably and reliably. The patient would plan to increase each exercise by a set amount each day or two. It is stressed that these quotas should be kept up irrespective of the patient's pain level. If a patient finds the rate of increase too difficult, they should set the daily quotas at a lower level and increase more slowly. The same planned and step-by-step approach is taken with other goal activities, such as walking, driving, return to work, reducing the use of medication, etc. For the patient who is often unable to perform necessary functions due to the unpredictable nature of the pain, this approach, by starting at an initially low level, can gradually enable desirable activities to be accomplished. This can be very reinforcing for the patient and can improve confidence considerably.

Typically, the operant approach has been employed in inpatient settings, where the multidisciplinary treatment staff can gain some control over reinforcement contingencies, particularly the differential reinforcement of desired goal activities and the non-reinforcement of pain behaviours.[8–10] However, the operant approach can be employed in outpatient settings, especially if the patient's spouse is able to participate in the implementation of the programme. Despite there being less control of the environment by the treatment staff in outpatient settings, patients can profitably set weekly activity and exercise goals which they carry out at home. Weekly clinic visits help to keep the programme on course, to sort out any problems, to reinforce achievements and to set new goals.[11]

The most suitable patients for the operant approach are those who have become very inactive due to their pain or exhibit a great deal of pain behaviour.[9] It has generally been found that suitable chronic pain patients who are treated in this way achieve substantial changes in their target behaviours, but particular attention is required to help them to maintain these changes once the programme is completed.[12-15] This can be achieved by such arrangements as careful planning and practice in dealing with likely post-treatment problems, regular check-ups with pain clinic staff (even by telephone), or regular visits to the general practitioner to review and reinforce progress.

Cognitive–behavioural treatment

This approach incorporates operant principles but places more emphasis on training the patient to monitor and to deal with unhelpful beliefs about pain and unhelpful reactions to pain. For example, it has been found that reactions (cognitions) which are overly negative and helpless are associated with heightened distress and functional impairment.[16,17] Similarly, some beliefs about pain, especially those which view it as a mystery, are associated with greater degrees of difficulty in coping with it.[18] The work of Turk,[19] and others,[20] has provided ways of helping chronic pain patients to tackle these reactions and beliefs.

In cognitive-behavioural treatment patients are asked to monitor their thoughts and feelings in relation to their pain—usually by keeping a brief diary. The therapist then assists the patient first to recognize any unhelpful reactions or beliefs and second, to develop ways of challenging and then changing them to more helpful responses. The patient is asked to practice these skills between sessions with the therapist and to report back to the therapist regularly, both to review progress and to refine the approach. Gradually, the patient develops a repertoire of skills for dealing with their pain and associated problems.

Typically, most cognitive-behavioural treatments also include many of the features of the operant approach, such as goal setting and the planned and gradual increase in activity levels.[13,19] In the cognitive-behavioural approach, however, while the therapist will reinforce the efforts made by the patient, they will also explicitly encourage the patient to reinforce themselves (with self-praise or small treats) and to attribute any improvements to their own efforts rather than to those of the therapist.[19] In practice, the operant approach is often quite similar, but it is usually not stated so explicitly. Cognitive-behavioural treatments may also include training in the use of distraction and relaxation techniques.[14,17]

While there is no clear research evidence that the cognitive-behavioural approach is more or less effective than the operant approach, it is the authors' experience that changing the way patients think about their pain plays an important role in the success of pain management programmes. Whether these changes need be achieved directly through cognitive therapy remains to be determined.[17] It could also be argued that operant programmes inevitably involve cognitive elements anyway.

Relaxation and biofeedback

Training chronic pain patients to relax has three main aims: (1) to assist with coping, by reducing anxiety and enhancing a sense of self-control; (2) to reduce muscle tension which may exacerbate pain; and (3) to improve the ability to sleep. No particular relaxation technique has been shown to be reliably better than any other, but some of the better results associated with relaxation were based on an approach to relaxation which emphasized the use of relaxation as a coping technique to be practised in stressful situations, rather than simply practicing it once or twice a day in calm surroundings.[21,22]

Biofeedback EMG training has also been used, with and without relaxation training, to reduce muscle tension and to enhance coping with pain.[23] While most findings have showed no real advantage for biofeedback over relaxation training alone, a recent study with chronic low back pain patients found biofeedback alone as effective as a cognitive-behavioural treatment programme.[24] However, this finding will require replication, particularly as it is not clear if it was related to the patient sample employed.

There is evidence that relaxation training has helped chronic pain patients to reduce pain intensity, improve sleep, and to reduce reliance on analgesics.[21] However, as the problems presented by pain patients tend to be quite complex and interrelated, it is recommended that relaxation training be included as one element of a pain management programme, rather than be used alone.[17]

Psychotherapy

While there are many forms of psychotherapy, the term normally refers to treatments derived from psychodynamic theories of personality. It usually involves a therapist providing support and helping a patient to make sense of particular problems or even life-long difficulties.[25] This can help the patient to work out possible ways of viewing and dealing with these problems.

Interventions of this nature have been found helpful to only a limited extent with chronic pain patients and much of the evidence is anecdotal in nature.[25] However, it is possible that psychotherapy may be more effective if combined with the more action-oriented behavioural approaches—for which there is far greater empirical support.

MODES OF DELIVERY

Psychological treatments can be provided in a number of ways. Inevitably, each has its advantages and disadvantages.

Individual versus group formats

The individual format

Patients may be seen individually by a psychologist or psychiatrist on a outpatient basis for varying lengths of time. Other family members may also be present at the treatment sessions. Other pain clinic staff, such as a physiotherapist or anaesthetist, would not normally be present, but may also have seperate sessions arranged with the patient for ongoing treatment. This is probably the most common mode of delivery of psychological treatments for chronic pain patients in Britain.

The advantages of this format include the opportunity to tailor the treatment more precisely to the assessed needs of the patient than may be possible in a group format. Furthermore, the facilities required are minimal (a small consulting room), and there is also the prospect of flexibility in number and timing of sessions. On the other hand, one of the disadvantages of the individual format, compared to the group format, is that there is no opportunity to utilize the experiences that the patient may share with other pain patients, which can be very helpful in creating an encouraging and supportive treatment environment. The individual format may also be less efficient than the group format in terms of the number of patients that can be seen in a limited time. While the opportunity to deal with a patient's problems in greater depth can be useful, it also runs the risk of continuing the treatment for longer than may be necessary. Although clear goals and an agreed treatment period can help to minimize this problem.

Unfortunately, while anecdotal accounts are available, there are no published studies examining in a critical fashion the outcome of individual psychological treatment for chronic pain.[26] This may not be surprising in the light of the individual aspects of any such treatment and the difficulties of undertaking such research in the usual clinical setting.

The group format

Typically, in outpatient settings, patients would be seen in groups of about 10 for fixed periods–often 8 to 10 weeks–on a weekly basis.[17,27] The sessions usually last from 1 to 3 hours and often involve more than one therapist during each session. For example, one part of the session may involve doing exercises with the physiotherapist, while other parts would focus on setting individual activity goals, relaxation practice, and discussion about pain management, etc. with a psychologist.[28]

The advantages of the group format are that not only does it capitalize on the encouragement and support of other patients, but also the participants can learn a great deal from each other, which can be very useful if managed effectively by the therapist. The group format also lends itself easily to the integration of psychological and physiotherapy treatments as they take place within the one session. While such an integration is also possible within the individual format, the logistics of employing a physiotherapist and a psychologist may be more easily arranged in a group format than in a series of individual sessions which will often be on different days. Furthermore, partly because the group approach is necessarily less able to deal very closely with specific issues raised by individual patients, it is correspondingly easier to set limits on both the content and the number of treatment sessions.

The disadvantages of the group format revolve mainly around the reduced sensitivity and ability to deal with the particular needs of individual patients, compared to the individual treatment approach. Furthermore, if the participants in group treatment are not carefully selected, there can be a problem with disruptive patients, who may, for example, have a vested interest in not improving. This can undermine the confidence of other patients in the treatment unless the issue is handled adroitly by the group leader. There may also be limited flexibility for the group approach, in terms of session times, which may not suit all patients, and clearly, a larger room will be required for providing a treatment in a group format.

Inpatient versus outpatient

This issue primarily concerns group programmes rather than individual approaches, which are usually conducted on an outpatient basis. Most of the early pain management programmes in the United States were developed in inpatient settings, often on physical rehabilitation or psychiatric wards.[7,23] Subsequently, outpatient programmes were established, initially on a research basis,[27] but later as normal clinical facilities.[29] In recent years the costs of inpatient programmes have lead to a swing towards more outpatient approaches. In some cases these may involve the patients staying at a hotel nearby the hospital and attending the programme for up to 8 hours a day for 3 to 4 weeks,[26] but in others it involves attending a clinic for one session a week for several weeks.[28]

Due to a lack of controlled trials, it is not clear whether inpatient treatment is more effective than outpatient treatment or vice versa. However, in the only large scale comparison study to have been published, Large and his colleagues found inpatient treatment slightly superior to outpatient treatment.[30] Clearly this will need replication, but there is a general impression that the inpatient approach is more appropriate for the more dysfunctional patients (who may find just getting to outpatient appointments is a problem), those who are more depressed, and those who are more dependent on medication.[26] It is also the authors impression that the less motivated patients are more likely to be helped in inpatient settings, if only because once admitted to the unit they do not have to make the decision before each session as to whether they will attend that day, as is the case for outpatient treatments. On the other hand, it is argued that maintaining the gains made is easier following outpatient treatment as the patients have been practising the exercises and strategies at home throughout the treatment period, whereas inpatients have to make this adjustment following discharge.[26] However, despite the intuitive appeal of this view, there is little research evidence for a differential level of maintenance between the two approaches, which is interesting given that the more dysfunctional patients tend to be treated in inpatient settings in the United States.[31] Not surprisingly, the costs of treatment are usually higher for inpatient compared to outpatient treatments, however, the actual amounts vary from country to country—for example, in Britain a 4-week inpatient programme costs about £1,600 per patient (Cost of INPUT programme, St Thomas' Hospital, 1989), whereas estimates of similar US programmes currently range between $12,000 and $20,000.

APPLICATION OF PSYCHOLOGICAL APPROACHES IN PAIN MANAGEMENT PROGRAMMES

Although group pain management programmes are usually run or supervised by psychologists, their efficacy can be enhanced by utilizing the skills of a multidisciplinary team comprising say, physiotherapist, nurse, occupational therapist, nurse and doctor. Such a team needs to be well versed in the psychological principles of the approach being used. Tables 2 and 3 give examples of typical in and out patient programmes. Most programmes contain some or all of the following elements:

Exercise

Supervised by a physiotherapist. A combination of general exercises to improve fitness, specific exercises relevant to the condition to build up individual muscle strength, and stretch. The importance lies in starting at a level the patient can easily tolerate, building up levels gradually, tabulating progress and rewarding achievements according to the operant approach.

Goal setting

Supervised by occupational therapist or psychologist. The identification of specific activity goals, such as walking for 30 minutes,

Table 2 A typical day on an inpatient pain management programme

8.30–9.30	Education session (e.g. on pain mechanisms, drugs, etc.)
9.30–10.00	Relaxation training (Discussion and practice, review of progress)
10.00–10.15	*Morning tea*
10.15–11.15	Physiotherapy (instruction in and practice of exercises)
11.15–12.15	Occupational Therapy (review of progress, set goals for next day)
12.15–13.15	*Lunch*
13.15–14.15	Free time (patients may work on goals or see staff individually)
14.15–15.30	Behavioural group (discussion and training in applications of cognitive and behavioural approaches to dealing with specific problems)
15.30–15.45	*Afternoon tea*
15.45–16.30	Physiotherapy (Exercise practice)
16.45	Feedback (patients see psychologist individually and review day and progress)

that the patient wishes to achieve and their breakdown into attainable steps.

Detoxification

Supervised by nurse and doctor. The withdrawal of inappropriate or excessive medications can be achieved by either (a) the gradual cutdown of tablets according to an agreed schedule, or (b) the use of a cocktail of morphine or methadone. Both methods appear to be effective.

Education

Pain patients often have a very poor idea of the nature of their illness and the physiology of pain. Conducted in an interactive way, discussions can clarify misunderstandings, dispell anxiety and explain perceived phenomena.

Cognitive therapy

Supervised by psychologist. The identification of thoughts and feelings regarding pain and the recognition and alteration of those that are unhelpful or inappropriate.

Table 3 Typical outpatient programme bases on 8–10 people attending for 3 hours once a week for 8 weeks. Staff: psychologist (ps), physiotherapist (pt), occupational therapist (ot), nurse (n), doctor (dr)

	time (h)		staff
week 1	1	introduction–model of chronic pain	ps
	1/2	start relaxation	ps
	1	start exercises (circuits)	pt
	1/2	goal setting: homework, long term goals	ot
week 2	1/4	review progress–reinforce achievements	ps
	3/4	education: disuse and healing	pt
	1	exercise & stretching and posture	pt
	3/4	goal setting: gradual increase & pacing concept	ot
	1/4	relaxation	ps
week 3	1/4	review progress–reinforce achievements	ps
	3/4	education: drugs and their effects & problems	n
	3/4	exercise & info. on muscles and joints	pt
	3/4	goal setting: further breakdown	ot
	1/4	introduction to thoughts and feelings	ps
	1/4	relaxation	ps
week 4	1/4	review progress–reinforce achievements	ps
	1	introduction to cognitions	ps
	1	exercises	pt
	1/2	goal setting: check medication reduction	ot
	1/4	relaxation	ps
week 5	1/4	review progress–reinforce achievements	ps
	3/4	cognitive concepts and applications	ps
	1/2	exercises & info, on slipped discs & X rays	pt
	1/2	goal setting	ot
	1	education: pain mechanisms and treatment	dr
	1/4	relaxation	ps
week 6	1/4	review progress–reinforce achievements	ps
	3/4	cognitive strategies and applications	ps
	3/4	goal setting: discharge planning, set backs	ot
	3/4	exercise	pt
	1/4	relaxation	ps
week 7	1/4	review progress–reinforce achievements	ps
	1	pain management–over view & set backs	ps
	3/4	exercise	pt
	1/2	goal setting	ot
	1/4	relaxation	ps
week 8	1/2	review progress–reinforce achievements	ps
	1/2	review maintenance and flare up plans	ps
	1/2	exercise	pt
	1/2	questions and answers	all
	1/2	passing out	all

Relaxation training

Supervised by psychologist or occupational therapist. Decreases muscle tension, improves sense of control of pain, relieves anxiety, aides sleep and may reduce pain.

Sleep

Attention to problems with sleep can be helpful for the many patients for whom this is a problem. Therapy involves the identification of inappropriate behaviours, decreasing anxiety, removing unhelpful pharmacotherapy, and teaching a relaxation technique.

Family involvement

One or more of the treatment staff should meet with a member of the patient's family to discuss and explain the programme, to identify any problems at home that may have a bearing on the successful outcome of the programme, and to advise the family on how they can help the pain patient. Sometimes it can be helpful to see the family member alone, but often the family and patient can be seen jointly.

EFFICACY OF PSYCHOLOGICAL TECHNIQUES USED IN PAIN MANAGEMENT

Very few of the multiplicity of treatments available for chronic pain have been adequately evaluated, and we must include psychological techniques in this generalization, although there is more supporting evidence for many of them than for many physical treatments. In particular the data examining the role of the single psychologist providing out patient treatment, either in isolation or in conjunction with conventional pain clinic treatments, is either anecdotal[26] or a series of individual cases reviewed together.[32] There is, however, a substantial body of literature concerning group behavioural interventions and pain management programmes for chronic pain states, mostly claiming the treatment to be helpful. While there are many methodological difficulties associated with such studies (see Table 4), there seems no doubt about the efficacy of many of the interventions. These studies have been comprehensively reviewed by Turner and Chapman[13] and more recently by Linton.[14,15] The interested reader is referred to these articles for a fuller assessment than is possible here.

In general studies have used a number of criteria for measuring change including the following:

Activity level

Studies have utilised a number of methods of measuring time spent resting, including sensors in beds. Operant programmes

Table 4   Problems associated with outcome research in chronic pain: confounding variables

Patient related problems	age
	sex
	diagnosis/site of pain
	pain severity
	duration of illness
	past history
Treatment related problems	duration
	components
	inpatient/outpatient
	staff mix
	expertize of staff
Study design	design
	numbers
	controls
	randomization
	measures used
Follow up	follow up interval
	duration of follow up
	methodology of follow (e.g. telephone)
	dropouts
Writing up	full description of treatment

have reported substantial increases in uptime and most measures of physical performance.[7,33,34]

Pain behaviour

Most programmes have reported decreases in pain behaviours such as groaning, limping, rubbing, bracing, talking about pain etc.[33,35]

Medication intake

Debate continues about the appropriateness of strong analgesia in chronic benign pain but few would dispute that function can be predjudiced by powerful analgesics, sedatives and tranquilizers. For this reason many behavioural programmes attempt to withdraw all or some of the patients' prescription drugs. Outcome data support the efficacy of such approaches.[21,35,36]

Return to work

Most patients attending pain management programmes are out of work and thus return to gainful employment would appear to be an attractive outcome measure. There are however many factors affecting work status other than pain, and thus this measure should not be viewed as a vital component of outcome data. Many programmes have nevertheless been successful at returning people to work.[10,37]

Mood

The mood of patients attending pain management programmes has been noted to improve in a number of studies. Maruta reported that patients treated in a pain management programme showed similar improvements in mood to a group treated with antidepressants.[38]

Pain level

It is perhaps surprising that programmes aimed at improving function should decrease pain but this has been reported in a number of studies.[35,39,40] However, this is not always the case and even when it occurs there is a suspicion that while it may be statistically significant, it may not be clinically significant. There are, however, insufficient data to predict which groups of patients will tend to achieve the greater pain reduction.

Utilization of medical resources and cost effectiveness

While this data is often difficult to obtain, some studies have reported decreased use of health care facilities following cognitive-behavioural treatment programmes.[41] The cost effectiveness of pain management programmes was considered by Steig[42] in a retrospective study. His conclusions were that substantial long-term savings could be made.

CONCLUSIONS AND RECOMMENDATIONS

Viewing complex chronic pain syndromes from a strict biomedical standpoint has insuperable limitations, and it remains unlikely that advances in neurobiology will ever explain all of the symptomatology about which patients complain. Conventional medical approaches are often unable to adequately treat many of these conditions, leading to frustration of both physician and patient. Behavioural medicine, in contrast, has demonstrated that many of the dysfunctions exhibited by patients with chronic pain can be viewed as learned phenomena which can be modified by psychological interventions. Psychological treatment can teach patients ways of improving their performance to bring enjoyable and necessary activities within the realm of everyday function. In addition, the transfer of the responsibility for the management of the illness to the patient, the application of cognitive strategies and the utilisation of relaxation techniques can considerably reduce the distress for the sufferer. For these reasons psychological approaches have a well established role in the treatment of chronic pain. These may be provided by psychiatrist or psychologist, however, all those involved in the treatment of chronic pain should be aware of the psychological aspects of chronic pain. Physicians referring patients for psychological treatment should ensure that they adequately prepare the patient for such treatment through full explanation and discussion.

Provision of integrated psychological services within pain clinics is often inadequate at present and must be improved if optimal treatment is to be provided. Preferably such services should be provided in a coordinated interdisciplinary manner.

REFERENCES

1 Engel GL. The need for a new medical model: a challenge for biomedicine. Science 1977; 196: 129–136
2 American Psychiatric Association, Diagnostic and statistical manual of mental disorders, 3rd edn., Washington DC.: A.P.A., 1980
3 Large RG. DSM III diagnoses in chronic pain: confusion or clarity? J Nerv Men Dis 1986; 174: 295–303
4 Merskey H. Traditional individual psychotherapy and psychopharmacotherapy In: AD Holzman, DC Turk (eds). Pain management. A handbook of psychological treatment approaches. New York: Pergamon, 1986
5 Cameron R, Shepel LF. The process of psychological consultation in pain management. In: AD Holzman, DC Turk (eds). Pain management. A handbook of psychological treatment approaches. New York: Pergamon, 1986
6 Turk DC, Holzman AD. Commonalities among psychological approaches in the treatment of chronic pain: specifying the meta-constructs. In: AD Holzman, DC Turk (eds). Pain management. A handbook of psychological treatment approaches. New York: Pergamon, 1986
7 Fordyce WE, Fowler R, Lehman J, DeLateur B, Sand P, Treischman R. Operant conditioning in the treatment of chronic pain. Arch Phys Med Rehabil 1973; 54: 399–408
8 Fordyce WE. Behavioural methods for chronic pain and illness. St. Louis: CV Mosby, 1976
9 Gil K, Ross SL, Keefe FJ. Behavioural treatment of chronic pain. Four pain management protocols. In: France RD. Krishnana KRR. Chronic pain Washington: American Psychiatric Press, 1988
10 Roberts AH, Reinhardt L. The behavioural management of chronic pain: long term follow up with comparison groups. Pain 1980; 8: 151–62

11 Hanson RW, Gerber KE. Coping with chronic pain: a guide to patient self management. Guildford Press: New York, 1990
12 Keef FJ. Behavioural assessment and treatment of chronic pain: current status and future directions. J Consult Clinic Psych 1982; 50: 363–75
13 Turner JA, Chapman CR. Psychological interventions for chronic pain: a critical review. Pain 1982; 13: 23–46
14 Linton SJ. A critical review of behavioural treatments for chronic benign pain other than headache. Br J Clin Psychol 1982; 21: 321–37
15 Linton SJ. Behavioural remediation of chronic pain: a status report. Pain 1986; 24: 125–41
16 Rosenteil AK, Keefe FJ. The use of coping strategies in chronic low back pain patients: relationship with patient characteristics and current adjustment. Pain 1983; 24: 33–44
17 Turner JA, Clancy S. Strategies for coping with chronic low back pain relationship to pain and disability. Pain 1986; 24: 355–364
18 Williams DA, Thorne BE. An empirical assessment of pain beliefs. Pain 1989; 36: 351–8
19 Turk DC, Meichenbaum D, Genest M. Pain and behavioural medicine: a cognitive behavioural perspective. Guildford: New York, 1983
20 Philips HC. The psychological management of chronic pain: a treatment manual. New York: Springer, 1988
21 Linton SJ, Gotestam KG. A controlled study of the effects of applied relaxation plus operant procedures in the regulation of chronic pain. Br J Clin Psychol 1984; 23: 291–9
22 Linton SJ, Melin L. Applied relaxation in the management of chronic pain. Behav Psychol 1983; 11: 337–50
23 Keefe FJ, Block AR, Williams RB, Surwit RJ. Behavioral treatment outcome of chronic low back pain: clinical outcome and individual differences in pain relief. Pain 1981; 11: 221–31
24 Schugens MM, Flor H. Cognitive behavioural treatment of chronic pain: a preventive study. Paper given at First International Congress of Behavioural Medicine. Upsala, Sweden 1990
25 Merskey, H. (1986) Traditional individual psychotherapy and psychopharmacology. In: AD Holzman, DC Turk (eds). Pain management. A handbook of psychological treatment approaches. New York: Pergamon, 1986
26 Holzman AD, Turk DC, Kerns RD. The cognitive-behavioural approach to the management of chronic pain. In: AD Holzman, DC Turk (eds). Pain management. A handbook of psychological treatment approaches. New York: Pergamon, 1986
27 Turner JA. Comparison of group progressive relaxation training and cognitive behavioural group therapy for chronic low back pain. J Consult Clin Psychol 1982; 52: 757–65
28 Skinner JB, Erskine A, Pearce S, Rubenstein M, Taylor M, Foster C. The evaluation of a cognitive behavioural treatment programme in outpatients with chronic pain. J Psychosom Res 990; 34: 1–7
29 Newman RI, Seres JL. The interdisciplinary pain centre: an approach to the management of chronic pain. In: AD Holzman, DC Turk (eds). Pain management. A handbook of psychological treatment approaches. New York: Pergamon, 1986
30 Peters JL, Large RG. A randomised controlled trial evaluating in and out-patient pain management programmes. Pain 1990; 41: 283–294
31 Kerns RD, Turk DC, Holzman AD, Rudy TE. Comparison of cognitive behavioural and behavioural approaches to the outpatient treatment of chronic pain. Clin J Pain 1986; 1: 195–203
32 Aronoff GM, Evans WO, Enders PL. A review of follow up studies of multidisciplinary pain units. Pain 1983; 16: 1–11

33 Cinciripini PM, Floreen A. An evaluation of a behavioural programme for chronic pain. J Behav Med 1982; 5: 575–89
34 Swanson D, Swenson W, Maruta T, McPhee M. Program for managing chronic pain. Mayo Clin Proc 1976; 51: 401–11
35 Miller C, LeLieuvre RB. A method to reduce pain in elderly nursing home residents. Gerontologist 1982; 22: 314–7
36 Lutz RW, Silbert M, Ohlson N. Treatment outcome and compliance with therapeutic regimens: long term follow up of a multidisciplinary pain program. Pain 1983; 17: 301–8
37 Gottlieb HJ, Koller R, Alperson BR. Low back pain comprehensive rehabilitation program: a follow up study. Arch Phys Med Rehabil 1982; 63: 458–60
38 Maruta T, Vatterot MK, McHardy MJ. Pain management as an antidepressant: long term resolution of pain associated depression. Pain 1989; 36: 335–7
39 Flor H, Haag G, Turk DC, Koehler H. Efficacy of EMG biofeedback pseudotherapy and conventional therapy for Chronic rheumatic back pain. Pain 1983; 17: 21–31
40 Large RG, Lamb AM. Electromyographic (EMG) feedback in chronic musculoskeletal pain a controlled trial. Pain 1983; 17: 167–77
41 Moore JE, Chaney EF. Outpatient group treatment of chronic pain: effects of spouse involvement. J Consult Clin Psych 1985; 53: 326–9
42 Steig RL, Williams RC, Timmermans-Williams G, Tafuro F, Gallagher LA. Cost benefits of interdisciplinary pain treatment. Clin J Pain 1986; 1: 189–193

British Medical Bulletin (1991) Vol. 47, No. 3, pp. 762–785

Pain clinics and pain clinic treatments

J C D Wells
Centre for Pain Relief, Walton Hospital, Liverpool

J B Miles
Department of Neurosciences, Walton Hospital, Liverpool

Chronic pain is multi-factorial, and consequently a multidisciplinary approach is essential for its proper management. Pain Clinics may treat acute pain, chronic pain and cancer pain, and need to differentiate between these different conditions. Careful diagnosis and assessment is essential, including history, examination, questionnaires and relevant investigations. A variety of treatments exist to manage chronic pain, some of which have already been discussed in this issue. Treatments may be summarized as drugs, surgical (including nerve blocks), stimulation techniques, psychological techniques and general or physical measures. If a *Pain Relief Unit* has the ability to provide all of these types of treatment, then it can manage any type of pain, with the ability to relieve pain and improve quality of life greatly in a significant number of sufferers.

The preceding chapters will have shown the complexities of both the aetiology and management of various types of pain. This should convince the reader of the necessity for specialized Units to be set up for the better management of patients with chronic pain. The idea of a *Pain Relief Clinic* is generally credited to J Bonica, as a result of his observations of soldiers in continuous severe pain as a result of battle injuries.[1] He became aware that it was impossible to properly treat these patients merely with the skills of one specialist, and that a multidisciplinary approach was essential in order to manage the various types of pain as successfully as possible. It took a considerable time to spread the word— lack of funding, lack of time and lack of understanding of the concept, all combining to prevent any rapid progress. However, gradually Pain Clinics appeared, some progressing to well-organized multidisciplinary units,[2] whilst others remained as small or single-modality treatment units. Pain Clinics have now been set up, and continue to be set up, worldwide. Their aims include the diagnosis and assessment of pain, treatment, teaching and training, evaluation of success rates and research into pain mechanisms and improved methods of treatment.

Three general types of pain can be considered—acute pain, chronic pain and cancer pain. The importance of acute pain, in particular post-operative pain, has recently been highlighted,[3] and its clinical management has been outlined by Justins & Richardson in this issue. Other chapters cover aspects of cancer pain and chronic pain. Three main classes of chronic pain can be considered. Firstly, there is pain that appears because of a specific acute injury or disease, but persists long beyond the normal healing time. Secondly, there is pain that is related to chronic disease, whether this is due to mechanical or degenerative factors such as arthritis, or to neurological conditions. Thirdly, there is pain which in the light of our present knowledge has no known organic cause.

Many doctors fail to differentiate clearly between acute and chronic pain, and use acute pain treatments to try to help chronic pain sufferers. They encourage rest and medications, which, whilst appropriate in a limited condition, lose their relevance in the chronic pain sufferer. These doctors often become frustrated or even angry because the patients do not get better, which sometimes destroys the doctor's confidence in his futile efforts to treat them. This sometimes leads to them accusing the patient of lying about the pain or imagining it. Very few patients with chronic pain are malingerers. None actually 'imagine' it. Pain is an emotional experience, and Sternbach has said, 'Pain is what the patient says it is, and exists wherever he says it does'.[4] The fact that it may be coming from emotional or psychological causes, as well as or rather than physical ones, means that the treatment methods employed should be slightly different, rather than the patient should be dismissed as a nuisance. In this issue, psychological factors have been considered by Main & Spanswick, and their management by Pither & Nicholas. We can now consider the aims of a Pain Clinic in more detail.

DIAGNOSIS AND ASSESSMENT OF PATIENTS WITH CHRONIC PAIN

Every effort should be made to establish a diagnosis before commencing treatment. A full history should be taken which includes the onset of the pain, its initial cause, its course in time, its nature, exacerbating or relieving factors, the pattern of the pain and what treatment modalities have already been attempted and with what results. Previous case records must be obtained prior to seeing the patient, even though these are often voluminous. A pain clinician must rely heavily on other Consultants' careful assessment as to the presence or absence of organic pathology, and its expected contribution to the patient's complaint. This can lead to errors via 2 routes:

1. Many patients arrive with an organic diagnosis which has been given to them as a 'tag' by a previous specialist, resident or General Practitioner. The patient may have been told a diagnosis, and this same diagnosis is backed up in the referral letter, or the letter may say that the patient has got little or no organic pathology. This latter status is obviously most confusing, as the patient is convinced that he has organic disease, when the previous specialist knows that he hasn't! It will then have to be explained to the patient exactly what the previous specialist has found, and what the extent of the organic disease is and its likelihood to be initiating any or part of the pain described. Even when organic disease has been detected by a previous specialist, and is said to be the cause of the patient's symptoms, sometimes this is quite clearly not the case. Figure 1 shows one patient referred with a diagnosis of 'spondylolisthesis at L4/5', with a pain chart showing constant severe pain throughout almost the whole of the body.

2. It is always possible to see a patient who has organic pathology that has not yet been diagnosed. An open mind has to be kept as to the possibility of the emergence of an organic condition, or the development of a new condition in a patient who has been attending the Clinic for some time. For instance a recent patient referred with back pain 'secondary to an epidural performed for the relief of pain in labour' turned out to have back and abdominal pain that came on after eating fatty meals, which responded very well to the removal of a gall bladder containing numerous gallstones!

Physical examination of the patient is essential, as this establishes confidence in the fact that the doctor is interested in the

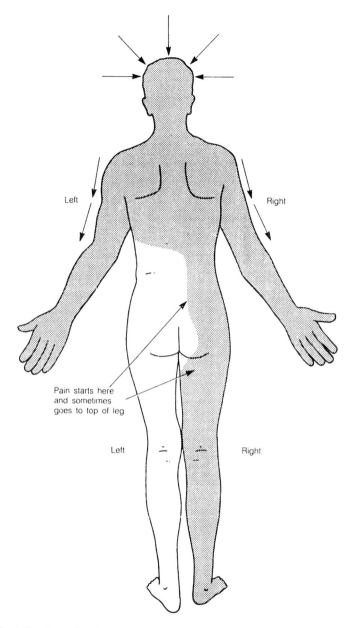

Fig. 1 Routine pain chart sent to all patients sometimes shows the disparity between any known organic disease and the patient's compaints. In this instance the patient was referred with a diagnosis of spondylolisthesis at L4–5. The patient has shaded in the areas of pain, with arrows showing the worst pains.

patient and believes his symptoms. Relevant investigations are also required in specific patients, although usually the patient has been well investigated prior to his attendance. Once all this has been done, an idea of the various factors contributing to the patient's chronic pain can be developed (*see* Fig. 2). It is important to be frank and direct with the patient as to the present state of knowledge of the organic pathology, and what symptoms it might be expected to cause. Even if the pathology does not completely explain the patient's symptoms, it should be stressed that these are believed, but that they may arise from other mechanisms such as muscle spasm or psychological factors, so that there are often several mechanisms contributing to the pain, all of which need an appropriate method of management.

We send out a complex questionnaire to the patient prior to his arrival at Clinic, which allows us to develop a useful profile on the patient and his pain state, and gives us valuable demographic data. A further questionnaire is completed at the time of the first consultation, and shorter follow-up questionnaires are completed on subsequent visits.[5]

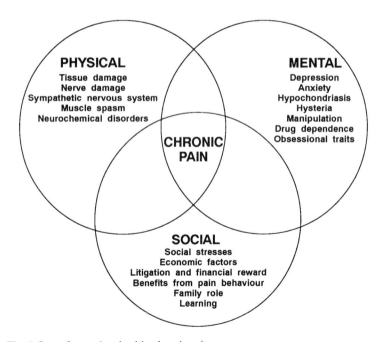

Fig. 2 Some factors involved in chronic pain.

Once the nature of the pain is fully understood, its effect on the individual is assessed. Sleep pattern, requirement for drugs and activities are all carefully noted. Activities include the amount of time the patient is up out of bed, sitting, standing and walking about, whether he can do various tasks relevant to his daily life, occupational history and social and sexual limitations caused by the pain. The described level of pain may be out of proportion to the activities, and if the activity level is reasonable, then the patient should not be over-treated. Sometimes activity levels are greatly reduced, with litle evidence of organic disease, and then the patient needs to be educated into returning to normal duties, without mechanistic intervention (as described by Pither & Nicholas in this issue).

Once the social and general history has been taken, examination includes not only assessment of the general condition and specific organic pathology, but also an assessment of any inappropriate illness behaviour (behaviour which is out of keeping with the known organic pathology) and the general psychological and social state of the patient.

Only when all of these factors have been considered and a multi-dimensional picture of the patient, his pain and his activity level have been built up, can any meaningful sort of treatment pro-gramme be planned. In many patients, all is still not clear after the initial interview, and subsequent investigations and assessment over a period of time need to be carefully planned in order for a full understanding to be developed. It must be remembered that however well the patients are assessed, and whatever the resources that can be concentrated on them, a significant number of patients will not respond to treatment. Their patterns of pain and social activity are so deeply ingrained or rewarded, that they are stuck with it. It should be explained to these sufferers that they have now reached a state where they have been fully investigated and assessed, and that there is no further useful treatment that can be applied. With limited resources it is important to do this, rather than to spend all one's efforts on a few really tough patients who will never improve, neglecting others who will benefit from the interventions that the Pain Clinic can offer.

THERAPIES FOR CHRONIC PAIN

A wide spectrum of therapies is currently available for the treat-ment of chronic pain, and the basic aim of the clinic is to select the most appropriate method or methods to carry them out and to review their efficacy. It must be explained to the patient and his family that in most cases a complete cure is unlikely, and that treatment will be aimed at achieving a reduction in pain and/or an increase in activities and improved quality of life.[6] Very occasionally, treatment of the underlying cause of the pain can be effected, although usually this is not the function of Pain Clinics and will already have been done by some other specialist, or the patient will need to be referred to some other specialist for a specific treatment. There are 5 general classes of therapy which are used in Pain Clinics. These can be classed as: (1) medical (drugs), (2) surgical (including nerve blocks), (3) stimulation techniques, (4) psychological intervention, and (5) general. These will now be considered in greater detail, with reference to the number of patients treated in our Unit and to the efficacy of these treatments (see Table 1), with general success rate at 3 months.

Medical treatments

Primary analgesic drugs (Table 2)

Many papers[7-9] have outlined the use of drug therapy in Pain Clinics. Because of their great importance, opiates have been discussed in great detail in this issue, particularly in cancer pain relief. However, they are not usually appropriate in the management of other chronic pain syndromes. Anti-inflammatory agents are not addictive, and can be helpful, but usually patients attending a Pain Clinic have already tried and failed with this type of therapy.[9] If a stronger agent than this is to be used, it must be ensured that the patient not only complains of less pain while on it, but that his activities have been increased and that this increase

Table 1 Treatments given at the first visit, their relative frequency and the success rates of these treatments when assessed at 3 months

Treatment	Proportion of patients receiving treatment (%)	Efficacy of therapy at 3 months (%)
Drugs	43	45
Blocks	26	45
Surgery	2	44
Stimulation Techniques	13	37
Psychological	14	47
Physical	2	30

Table 2 Primary analgesics in common usage

1. Non-steroidal anti-inflammatory agents
   e.g. Paracetamol
   Ibuprofen
   Indomethacin

2. Low-potency opioid agents
   e.g. Codeine
   Dextropropoxyphene
   Dihydrocodeine

3. Potent Opioids (*see* McQuay and Hanks in this issue)

4. Other analgesic drugs
   e.g. Nefopam (Acupan)
   Meptazinol
   Tramadol

is maintained. Otherwise the effect of the drug is merely to convert the patient from one who is doing nothing and complaining, to one who is doing nothing and not complaining. Many patients attending Pain Clinics on opiate derivatives like dihydrocodeine, dextropropoxyphene and codeine, or who are taking sedatives and tranquillizers on a regular basis, have to be withdrawn from their medication before any progress can be made with treatments.[10]

Nefopam is a moderately strong analgesic, which is not related to the non-steroidals. It is not addictive, although it may cause drowsiness and nausea. Meptazinol is a centrally-acting analgesic with agonist and antagonist properties. It does not produce respiratory depression, and has a lower abuse potential. Tramadol is a drug not available in the United Kingdom, although it has been used for many years in Germany and is now the subject of interest. It is claimed to be almost as powerful as opiates, without opiate side-effects.[11]

Secondary analgesic drugs

Many other drugs are available which have the ability to relieve pain, but which are used primarily for some other property. They have been termed 'secondary analgesics'.[8] Their usefulness in the treatment of acute pain is very limited, but they do have value in the treatment of chronic pain, and they may be classified according to their primary therapeutic mode of action.

Psycho-active drugs. The following types of drugs can be considered: antidepressants, anticonvulsants, tranquillizers, hypnotics. Many patients attending Pain Clinics have mood changes, and it may be thought that these drugs are given for this reason. However, many appear to have intrinsic analgesic properties of their own, and when used in appropriate situations can produce a striking response.

(a) *Antidepressants*. Chronic pain patients are often depressed, either as a cause or a consequence of their pain. However, some who do not appear to be depressed can get pain relief from these agents on small dosages. The onset of this analgesic effect may occur in about 3–7 days, which is more rapid than the antidepressant effect, which usually takes 14 days to occur. It has been suggested that the analgesic and antidepressant action of tricyclics and monoamine-oxidase inhibitors are caused by their action on neurotransmitter function, particularly those mediated by classical amine and indoleamine systems.[12] All of the tricyclics inhibit presynaptic re-uptake of noradrenaline, and produce changes in the sensitivity of pre- and post-synaptic receptors. Monks[13] reviewed 48 papers describing 52 trials, with a wide range of disorders covered. Most of these trials were of inadequate design; however, 17 were double-blind and in every case (except for 2 of 3 trials on low back pain) good effects were shown. A long-term trial of 104 patients with no significant somatic findings[14] showed a 57% improvement from 9 to 16 months, with 31% having been withdrawn from treatment because of side-effects or lack of efficacy. Hanks[15] concluded that they did have a part to play, but were probably over-used. Treatment outcomes observed in our own Unit confirmed this—only 15% of patients treated with antidepressants had long-term benefit, 10% had a short-term improvement, 63% remained the same and 12% actually got worse. Amitriptyline appears as effective as any, and the dose needs to be titrated for the individual patient, starting at 25 mg at night, and increasing every 5 days if tolerated, or even reducing the dose to 10 mg (*see* Bowsher, this issue).

(b) *Anticonvulsants*. Trousseau described certain types of pain as epileptiform or neuralgia over 100 years ago. Any shooting or stabbing pain may be so described. Anticonvulsants were first used for trigeminal neuralgia in the 1940s,[16] and they may also be effective in a wide range of other painful conditions (*see* Bowsher, this issue). All of these drugs have side-effects, and these must be recognized before embarking on therapy. They tend to produce drowsiness if introduced rapidly, and need to be started at low doses and gradually increased. We find carbamazepine particularly sedating and the least well-tolerated by patients. It is introduced at a dosage of 100 mg twice a day, and increased gradually to a maximum of 1600 mg, which is sometimes needed for the control of trigeminal neuralgia. Recently, we have used oxcarbazepine, with an apparent reduction in the incidence of side-effects. Both drugs can produce drowsiness, ataxia, dizziness, visual and intestinal disturbance and a generalized erythematous rash. Blood dyscrasias can occur with carbamazepine.

Diphenylhydantoin, phenytoin and sodium valproate, are also used as anticonvulsants. Since the former can cause depression, it is infrequently used in our Unit. Sodium valproate appears to be better tolerated by most patients and is our drug of choice for initial treatment in shooting neurogenic pain, apart from trigeminal neuralgia. Follow up of our patients shows a much higher rate of success when anticonvulsants have been used for this type of pain, than when anti-depressants have been used for neurogenic pain in general. Patients on anticonvulsants show a long-term improvement in 48%, short-term improvement in 10% and worsening of the situation in only 6%.

(c) *Sedatives and tranquillizers.* All of these drugs are habituating, and their beneficial effect tends to wear off rapidly.[9] Thus they can only be used for a short time while positive steps are being taken in the way of anxiety management, relaxation training and improvement of sleep pattern. Whilst we continue to use benzodiazepines when the patient is already established on them, partly because it is difficult to wean them off, we virtually never initiate their usage in chronic pain.

Muscle relaxant drugs

Increased muscle tone is associated with many chronic pain conditions, and is accepted as the underlying cause in conditions such as tension headache and myofascial syndromes. Severe spasm may follow minor trauma, and may be reduced by limited courses of tranquillizers. Certain specific muscle relaxants have been tried, including orphenadrine (30 mg three times a day) and methocarbamol (1.5 mg daily). They inhibit repetitive segmental interneuronal discharges into the cord, and may often be found in preparations in combination with simple analgesics. Severe muscle spasm and contracture may be present in neurological syndromes, such as multiple sclerosis and polyneuritis. Dantrolene in a dosage of 25 mg a day, and baclofen commencing with 5 mg three times a day and increasing to 20 mg three times a day, have been used for this type of spasm. Good results sometimes accrue, but in general the results have been disappointing, there either being little effect or toxicity prevents continuation of the drug.

Adrenergic blocking agents

There are 3 areas in which these types of drug are particularly appropriate:

(a) *Facial pain*. Certain types of neuralgia appear to respond to propanolol in a dosage of 5 mg twice a day, increasing to a maximum of 50 mg twice a day. This is thought to have a quinine-like effect on the cell membrane.

(b) *Migraine*. This is accepted as being partially due to sero-tonin, and anti-serotonin agents have been used as a prophylactic measure. These include cyproheptadine, 2 mg four times a day, pizotifen, 0.5 mg three times a day and also clonidine, 0.025 mg daily, has had good effect in some patients.

(c) Reflex sympathetic dystrophy and causalgia (*see* Charlton, this issue).

Steroids

These can be used in many conditions, by many different routes. Their use in malignant disease has been discussed by Hanks (this issue) and obviously they are often used in inflammatory joint disease. The use of steroids in the epidural and subdural spaces is a well-recognized way of improving many chronic pain conditions, such as low back pain, and they can be injected into the joints to produce pain relief in the short term. However, there is evidence to suggest that this speeds up the eventual degeneration of an inflamed joint.

Other drugs

Many other drugs have been used, such as enzyme-blocking agents (e.g. D-lucine), transmitter precursors (e.g. L-tryptophan) and various peptides. Although they show promise for the future, as yet there is little general advice that can be given as to their usage, and they must remain as experimental agents at the present time.[7]

Surgical treatments

Nerve blocks

Peri and post-operatively, pain can be relieved by nerve blocks on a temporary basis, often with excellent results. It is tempting for the anaesthetist to think that a more permanent block will achieve just as good permanent results with chronic pain. However, permanent damage to nerves leads to both obvious and less obvious sequelae. There will often be damage to sensory and motor fibres, with an unpleasant lack of sensory input, or even worse, lack of movement. Secondly, even if weakness and paralysis can be avoided, damage to nerve tissue leads to central nervous system changes, which may sooner or later be evidenced as a neurological pain syndrome. An unpleasant and disabling dysaesthetic or phantom pain may occur in the original area, and experience has shown this to be largely untreatable. A full knowledge of the possible consequences of long-term neuronal blockade is essential before any such major and irreversible steps are taken.[17] Pain relieving techniques have been given a bad name in the past because of inappropriate procedures carried out on a patient whose pain is multi-factorial and not completely assessed. However, in the correct situation, some permanent nerve blocks can give excellent results.[18-20]

Diagnostic blocks

These may fulfil 3 functions. Firstly, by blocking off selective pathways, they may add to the assessment of factors influencing the pain. Secondly, the prognosis for more permanent blockade can be elicited. Also, in chronic pain, the mere interruption of a pain pathway for a few hours can sometimes result in long-term pain relief. The diagnostic block can be combined with a further therapeutic agent, for example steroids, usually in a prolonged-release form such as depo-Medrone (methylprednisolone), or guanethidine for sympathetic blockade. Whilst these substances do not produce long-term nerve block, they sometimes appear to achieve long-term pain relief. There is a great deal of controversy as to whether these agents actually do promote any improvement in results, and carefully controlled clinical trials are still needed to assess whether adding guanethidine in the Hannington-Kiff technique[21] has any long-term physiological effect.

Depo-Medrone contains ethylene glycol as a preservative, and at present there are unsubstantiated claims in Australia that this causes arachnoiditis. Even though there is no evidence to support this, the Australian Defence Unions will not cover doctors who are using this substance in the epidural space. Consequently, although we have no qualms about the safety record of depo-Medrone, which we have used for years without ill-effect, we now use Kenalog in order to spare our patients trauma should 'scare stories' about depo-Medrone ever emerge in the press here.

Diagnostic blocks include paravertebral, intercostal and trigeminal blocks, facet nerve and facet joint injections for back pain, local infiltration, sympathetic blockade and differential spinal blockade. The idea of the latter is to give increasing concentrations of local anaesthetic into the cerebro-spinal fluid to achieve, (in order), sympathetic, sensory and motor blockade. Initially normal saline is given, to see if the patient appears to respond to placebos, and then different concentrations of lignocaine to produce graded blockade. If pain is still present after this, it must be assumed that the pain is central, and certainly not amenable to direct attacks upon the peripheral nervous system.[22] If diagnostic blocks confirm the likelihood that nerve pathways can be interrupted more permanently, then several ways exist of producing a long-term effect, although discussion of this is outside the scope of this chapter.[17,23,24] Table 3 shows results and comparisons of various types of block over the last 5 years.

Epidurograms

Gabor Racz has suggested that some patients have filling defects in the epidural space, when Omnipaque or Niopam is injected to

Table 3 Results and comparisons of various types of blocks over the last 5 years

	Improved	Short term improvement	Same	Worse (%)
Epidurals	20	28	50	2
Facet joint injection	9	21	62	8
Sympathectomy:				
L.A.	8	31	58	2
Chemical	40	25	26	9
Trigeminal:				
L.A.	18	34	42	6
Radiofrequency	82	3	5	10

Improvement is assessed on reduction in visual analogue scale, increase in activity and cessation of drugs, with the first column showing improvement at 3 months; 'short term improvement' means any significant increase in activity or in reduction of pain or analgesics outline this. This might indicate the presence of fibrous tissue which might impinge upon the nerve roots passing through the space, and consequently irritate them. Over the last 4 years we have carried out epidurograms in this way, and it is our experience that in those patients studied a significant number (54%) have a filling defect, which often correlates with the side and the neuronal level of the pain. Either the injecting needle, or a catheter passed through this needle, is then manipulated into the area shown, and a mixture of local anaesthetic, steroids and Hyalase (1500 units) is injected. Subsequent repeat blocks will show if there has been any resolution of the filling defect, as often improvement in the X-ray appearance correlates with pain relief. The benefits of epidural blocks have increased from 36 to 54% in our Unit since this technique was introduced.

More permanent procedures

The most successful destructive blocks are the radiofrequency lesion for trigeminal neuralgia, and percutaneous cordotomy for types of cancer pain not responsive to medication, as described by Hanks' in this issue. This gives 85% of our patients[19] good relief of pain, with low morbidity.[25,26]

Some destructive treatments have now been largely discontinued in our Unit. This includes facet rhizotomy, or facet joint denervation, which does not have any advantage over facet joint and facet nerve injections with local anaesthetic and steroids. The procedure is tedious for both patient and operator, with a significant morbidity, and is indeed now rarely used. Likewise, pituitary alcohol injection[27] is now recognised by most authorities as a major procedure with uncertain efficacy and unpleasant side-effects, and has largely been discontinued as a mechanism for managing cancer pain.

Operative techniques

Anterolateral cordotomy can be carried out by an open surgical approach, but as the results of percutaneous radiofrequency lesions are as good, this technique is reserved for those patients who are unable to lie still, or whose anatomy is so distorted that a percutaneous technique cannot be carried out.[28] Another form of surgical treatment which has been popular in the 80s is the dorsal route entry zone (DREZ) destruction. This has been used for some benign persisting pain syndromes, for instance the boundary dysaesthetic pain sometimes encountered in paraplegic patients. This has also been used for post-herpetic neuralgia. Enthusiastic proponents of this technique claim good success rates, but it is certainly a procedure where the assessment of the patient assumes great importance, and experience of the operator is essential.[28]

The most common neurosurgical procedure for pain in our Unit is microvascular decompression of the trigeminal ganglion for trigeminal neuralgia.[29] This appears to have a lower morbidity rate than the radiofrequency lesion, in that patients do not suffer with numbness or dysaesthetic pain (anaesthesia dolorosum) after the procedure. It is also longer lasting. We reserve this technique for younger patients, and those with first division trigeminal neuralgia, as radiofrequency destruction here produces a high level of ophthalmic complications. Other techniques, such as the use of glycerol or balloon catheters, have not been as effective as surgery or radiofrequency lesions in our hands.

Other surgical procedures for the relief of pain have been outlined, although they fall beyond the scope of most Pain Relief Clinics.[28,30]

Stimulation techniques

Acupuncture

Texts on acupuncture date back to at least 300 years B.C.. Acupuncture has been used as a treatment for many conditions, but appears to be most appropriate for the relief of acute pain, and it has been possible to perform surgery under acupuncture analgesia, initially in China. It has also been used in animals, and is now used widely by clinicians and indeed non-medical practitioners, for the treatment of chronic pain. There exists a great deal of conflicting scientific data on its mode of action and efficacy, but it does seem that there is an inherent analgesic action, which may well be due to A delta fibre stimulation.[31] As it is a simple and cheap treatment, with a very low incidence of side-effects, it must deserve a place in the treatment of chronic pain, and in particular in those patients with definite organic findings where nothing else seems to be of benefit.[32] It needs to be performed on a regular basis, as there is a finite length of action of effect for various patients, and it rarely produces a cure. Unfortunately at present there are few resources in the Health Service for regular acupuncture analgesia, even though this might well be a cost-effective form of treatment. Many Pain Clinics employ at least one person with a passing knowledge of acupuncture treatment, who can provide a useful service for some patients.

Electrical stimulation

Like many things in medicine, electrical nerve stimulation is not new, but a re-discovery of long-known principles. Naturally-generated electricity, for instance in the torpedo fish, was used to relieve types of chronic pain by the application of the fish to the painful part of the patient! There it produced a numbing sensation, thus relieving the pain. Hand-generated electricity was used to relieve pain and cure diseases in the 19th century, for instance by Sarlandier for rheumatism, but it was not until the description of the Gate Control Theory by Melzack and Wall in 1965[33] that doctors really accepted that there was a physiological explanation as to its efficacy. Initially transcutaneous electrical nerve stimulation was used to assess whether patients might benefit from dorsal column stimulation,[34] when it was noted that a significnt number of patients preferred this to the actual implant of a dorsal column electrode.

One or more pairs of electrodes are placed on the skin of the patient in the vicinity of the pain. A current is generated by use of a simple battery, provoking paraesthesia in the area of pain, and for the best response the paraesthetic tingling must mix in with the pain, and must itself prove a pleasant substitute for that pain. Conventional TENS is a low-intensity, high-frequency electrical message, but machines can be used as a high-intensity, low-frequency stimulator, so an acupuncture-like effect can be achieved. In many Pain Clinics the patient is instructed into the usage of the machine, and then loaned a unit to take home for a period of time to assess treatment efficacy. The more time that is spent going over the technique with the patient, the more likely it is to have a useful effect. Unfortunately, usually the patient will have to purchase his own machine if it is of benefit, at a cost of some £80 upwards. Many patients do purchase TENS machines, and get benefit from them for a significant period. Woolf has summarized the reported differential specificity for the different types of electrical stimulation.[35]

Dorsal column stimulation (DCS)

Spinal cord stimulation was applied to humans in pain within 2 years of the Gate Control Theory, in 1967.[34] Implanted stimulators were tried for a wide variety of pains and have proved successful in many types of pain, but only in a proportion of the sufferers. The method has been most readily applied to chronic pain associated with non-malignant conditions, particularly sufferers of chronic back and leg pain.

Assessment as to suitability for this treatment is difficult, but absolutely essential to attempt. Failure to relieve pain after surgical implantation is a further physical and psychological insult to the chronic pain sufferer. Also, the equipment is expensive and time-consuming for both patient and therapist. Assessment includes pharmacological, psychological and physiological scrutiny, and a trial percutaneous stimulation with an in-dwelling wire is used in all cases in our Unit.[36]

Back and leg pain sufferers constitute a potentially inexhaustible supply of candidates for this treatment, and those patients with leg pain with a minimal level of neurological deficit are those most likely to respond. Pain relief from successful implant can fade with time[37] but can also persist for more than 15 years.[38]

Deep brain stimulation (DBS)

This method has proved popular and effective in parts of North America, but in the United Kingdom patients are more resistant to the idea of cerebral implantation for non-life threatening conditions. A stereotactic technique is used to implant an electrode into the thalamus or medial lemniscus tract, but once again, thorough assessment of the likelihood of success has to be made, prior to embarking on this expensive and time-consuming method of treatment.

Psychological techniques

These have been covered by Main & Spanswick and Pither & Nicholas (this issue). Our own experience with a psychologically-orientated rehabilitation programme has been to convince us that this is an essential part of all Pain Relief Units. Our own Programme[23] has been running since 1982, and nearly 1000 patients have commenced the 4-week treatment. It has been possible to reduce the drug intake by 50%, to double the activity level of more than half of the patients and return 29% of those in the job market to work, in spite of an average length of time off work of 2.7 years prior to attendance on the Programme. It is our belief that even the most basic of Pain Relief Units should have some sort of rehabilitation programme employing the services of a psychologist or psychiatrist. This, combined with some form of exercise programme and relaxation training, seems the very minimum. It can be done on the basis of a half-day a week, over a regular period, probably almost as effectively as the ongoing programmes described by Pither and ourselves.

Our Programme is a 4-week course with patients attending every day from Monday to Friday, and with 2 new patients starting every week and joining a group which thus totals 8. Patients in their last week are expected to offer help to the new ones, improving compliance of both new patients and those who are completing their rehabilitation. We have found it important to set up a self-help group for patients who have completed the Programme, who are subsequently discharged from clinic once assessment of their progress following the course has been made. Our ex-patients have now set up a charity, *Self Help In Pain*, and are actively looking to expand this throughout the country. They envisage being able to support the setting up of peripheral units attached to other Pain Clinics in the future, and there is also the possibility of fund-raising for ongoing research into chronic pain and its treatment. This group has been formed for 7 years, although it is only during the last 2 years that significant growth has begun to occur. Those readers interested in further information on this subject should write to *Mrs B Cross, Secretary, SHIP, Room 27 (Old Sewing Room), Walton Hospital, Rice Lane, Liverpool L9 1AE.*

General measures

Many general measures exist to try and improve the lot of the chronic pain sufferer. These include improving the general health, the diet and environment of the patient and physical methods, such as vibration and massage. Application of heat or cold is often useful. Manipulation, whether by physiotherapeutic methods, osteopathic or chiropractic, may all have benefits for some patients. Alternative medicine, or perhaps we should say complementary medicine, also has an effect on chronic pain. Whilst acupuncture and chiropractice have both been shown in control trials to be effective, homeopathy, herbalism and healing seem interesting areas where the case is not yet proven.[39] Many ancient civilisations have practised interesting techniques for the promotion of good mental and physical health, and these can often be effective for those patients who wish to make a genuine effort to improve. This includes yoga and T'ai Chi. In both of these disciplines, as well as in the Moslem ritual of praying to Mecca, there is a good deal of regular physical activity, coupled with relaxation, and the importance of mental control over the body. This is certainly one of the most important aspects of the Pain Programmes now being slowly introduced in the United Kingdom.

SPECIFIC PAIN SYNDROMES

Many different types of patient with many different types of pain are seen in Pain Relief Units, but certain syndromes are seen regularly, some representing conditions which are difficult to treat with any success, while some are best managed by the multi-disciplinary approach adopted by Pain Clinics. Some of the most important of these are discussed briefly here.

Back pain

As outlined in the introduction, this is a major health problem. Contributing factors such as disc disease, facet joint disease, spondylolisthesis and arachnoiditis, must be identified and treated as fully as possible.[40] Muscle spasm plays a major role in adding to the pain and discomfort of chronic back disease. This spasm sometimes continues long beyond the healing of the original injury and may produce localized trigger points. Obviously the spasm and trigger points can be exacerbated by emotional stress, or even initiated by them. Psychological factors have been fully covered by Main & Spanswick and Pither & Nicholas (this issue). Our experience is that these are undoubtedly the most important issues in chronic back pain sufferers. A very high proportion of patients on our Pain Management Programme have chronic back and/or leg pain, and of all of the individual treatment groups at the Clinic, this is the most effective with a 47% improvement at 3 months. Taken in conjunction with other treatments which can be applied to back pain sufferers, there is an overall 68% of patients who get sustained increase in activities following treatment. This does depend on good resources, a multi-disciplinary team and a variety of different treatments.[41]

Myofascial pain

This used to be known as fibrositis, but tends to be rather ignored in the United Kingdom. Patients have specific areas of tenderness (trigger points) and pressure on these produces diffuse pain, increasing gradually in intensity, and spreading in various well-described patterns. This type of pain often begins at the time of a nerve injury, or a repetitive activity. Whilst some feel that the disease is due to increased muscle tension, others now regard this as a decrease in the microcirculation of muscle and tissue.[42] Myofascial syndromes may be secondary to an underlying pathology such as osteoarthritis, or be associated with clear psychological factors. A combination of physical and psychological factors should be used to improve the lot of the myofascial pain sufferer.

Malignant pain

Treatment of malignant pain is very different to that of chronic, non-malignant pain, or indeed acute pain. The patient is often aware that the pain indicates failure to treat the tumour successfully, and that the pain will continue until his death. He understandably becomes very dependent on his medical attendants. Although the tools are available to treat cancer pain successfully, they tend to be poorly used. In this issue McQuay and Hanks have outlined the use of opiate drugs, and indeed other therapies where these are not appropriate. Once again, a careful assessment of the patient is essential, and the multi-disciplinary team important, even if this means having ready access to other specialists for their own particular opinion.

Apart from drugs, the 2 techniques we have found most useful for the management of difficult cancer pain are drug delivery systems and the cordotomy. We use drug delivery systems where the pain is morphine-responsive, but the patient has unacceptable side-effects. A catheter is inserted percutaneously into the epidural or intrathecal space under aseptic technique, and is tunnelled anteriorly to an appropriate site over bone, for example the anterior aspect of the ribs, where it is connected to a reservoir. This reservoir is inserted into a subcutaneous pouch fashioned over this bony area.[42]

The system can then be topped up at regular intervals by nursing staff, or even by the patient or his relatives, or a constant infusion can be given for some pain sufferers. Intrathecal dosing in this way allows a dose of some 1/50th or 1/100th of the oral dose, with a greatly-lessened side-effect profile.[43] This is over and above that which might be achieved by keeping a constant blood level with a subcutaneous infusion. Also, as well as using morphine, we have recently used combinations with local anaesthetic and some of the neuropeptides, with good results. More recently we have been looking at the effect of morphine-6-glucuronide on cancer pain. This is a metabolite of morphine, and it appears to be at least 4 times as effective as an analgesic. That in itself may not be particularly remarkable, but in certain patients the therapeutic dose has been associated with even fewer side-effects, and it appears to merit further investigation.

The percutaneous cordotomy has already been mentioned in this chapter. It is particularly useful for unilateral cancer pain, especially if this is intermittent, when it is difficult to achieve an effective control of medication. Accurate diagnosis of the cause of the pain, specific appropriate therapy, with regular review, and support of the patient on an emotional and spiritual level, can achieve pain relief in over 97% of these patients.[17]

Other pain syndromes

Sympathetic pain, nerve injury, post-herpetic neuralgia, phantom limb pain, thalamic pain and trigeminal neuralgia have all been described in this issue (see Charlton and Bowsher). These conditions are so common, and their treatments so variable, that considerable space has been devoted to them. Further and better understanding of their causes, by means of basic scientific research, is gradually helping to build up appropriate treatment strategies.

CONCLUSION

Chronic pain is a debilitating and degrading condition. Its aetiology is largely multi-factorial, and only proper appreciation of the various factors which can combine to produce the patient's discomfort will allow effective treatment. The cost of pain to the country, the community and the pain sufferers themselves, is immense. The resource allocation specifically for chronic pain in the United Kingdom is pathetic, and increased resources to properly-funded multi-disciplinary Pain units would almost certainly be extremely cost-effective, reducing sickness benefits, insurance payouts and costly but inappropriate treatments elsewhere within the Health Service.

Money needs to be spent on research into the causes and treatment of chronic pain, and both medical students and doctors need to be taught more about chronic pain, and the difference between it and acute pain must be stressed. If in the proposed new Health Service in the United Kingdom, money were truly to follow patients, then with 11% of the population being in chronic pain, a massive amount of Pain Clinic development would take place. However, due to administrative bureaucracy, this is most unlikely to happen without a great deal of effort from all of the doctors involved in the treatment of chronic pain, and all of those chronic pain sufferers who require better and more comprehensive treatment.

REFERENCES

1 Rovenstine EA, Wertheim HM. Present status of regional anaesthesia. NY St J Med 1942; 42: 123–130
2 Newman RI, Painter JR, Seres JL. A therapeutic milieu for chronic patients. J Human Stress 1978; 4: 8–12
3 Cousins MJ. Acute Pain and the injury response: Immediate and prolonged effects. Regional Anaesthesia 1989; 14: 162–178
4 Sternbach RA. Pain patients, traits and treatment. New York: Academic Press, 1974
5 Cossins L. Features of commonest diagnoses in 1017 successive Pain Clinic cases. Pain 1990; (Suppl. 5): S75
6 Boulton TB. Editorial Anaesthesia 1978; 33: 225–226
7 Budd K. Pain. Update Postgraduate Series, Update Publications, 1984
8 Budd K. Analgesic Drugs. In: Williams NE, Wilson H (eds). Pain and its management. Int. Encyc. Pharmacology and Therapeutics, Section 112. New York: Pergamon Press, 1983; pp. 51–64
9 Melzack R, Wall PD. A textbook of pain. Edinburgh: Churchill Livingstone. 1984, pp. 505–537
10 Orme M, Graham-Jones S. The self-help guide. London: Penguin Books, 1988; pp. 106–109
11 Forth W, Martin E, Peter K. The relief of pain. Hoechst Medication Update; p 48
12 Wells JCD. The place of the pain clinic. In: Clinical Rheumatology. London: Bailliere, Volume 1, Part I, 1987, pp. 123–153
13 Monks RC. The use of psychotropic drugs in human chronic pain: A review. VIth World Congress of International College of Psychosomatic Medicine. Montreal, Canada, September 15th, 1981
14 Blumer D, Heilbronn M. Second year follow-up study on systematic treatment of chronic pain with antidepressants. Henry Ford Hospital Med Journ 1981; 29: 67–68

15 Hanks GW. Antidepressants in chronic Pain: A clinical perspective. In the pain clinic II. Utrecht: VNV Science Press, 1987, pp. 93–108

16 Crill W. Carbamazepine. Ann Intern Med 1973; 79: 79–80

17 Wells JCD. The use of nerve destruction for the relief of pain in cancer: A review. Palliative Med 1989; 3: 239–247

18 Wells JCD, Hardy PAJ. Continuous intrathecal lignocaine infusion analgesia: A case report of a 9-week 'spinal'. Palliative Med 1989; 3: 23–25

19 Wells JCD, Lipton S, Lahuerta J. Percutaneous cervical cordotomy: Results and complications in a recent series. Ann R Coll Surg Engl 1985; 67: 41–44

20 Loeser JD. Tic doloureux and atypical facial pain. In: Melzack R & Wall TD, eds. Textbook of pain. Edinburgh: Churchill Livingstone, 1984, pp. 426–434

21 Hannington-Kiff JG. Antisympathetic drugs in limbs. In: Melzack R & Wall PD, eds. Textbook of pain. Edinburgh: Churchill Livingstone 1984, pp. 566–573

22 Winnie AP, Collins VJ. The pain clinic I: Differential neuronal blockade in pain syndromes of questionable aetiology. Med Clin N Am 1968; 52: 123

23 Wells JCD. The place of the pain clinic. In: Clinical Rheumatology. London: Bailliere, Volume 1, Part 1, 1987, pp. 123–153

24 Swerdlow M. Current ideas on the place of nerve blocks in the treatment of chronic pain. In: The pain clinic II. Utrecht: VNV Science Press, 1987, pp. 159–166

25 Lipton S. Percutaneous electrical cordotomy in the relief of intractable pain. Br Med J 1968; 2: 210–212

26 Tew JM (Jr). Treatment of trigeminal neuralgia by percutaneous rhizotomy. In: Youmans JR, Neurological Surgery. London: Saunders, 1982, pp. 3564–3579

27 Wells JCD, Lipton S. Pituitary ablation for pain relief in cancer. Reviews on Endocrine-related Cancer 1984; 19: (Suppl 11) 11–15

28 Sweet WH, Poletti CE. Operations in the brain stem and spinal Canal (Appendix on 'Open Cordotomy'). In: Melzack R & Wall PD. Textbook of Pain, 1984, pp. 615–631

29 Janetta PJ. A microsurgical approach to the trigeminal nerve for tic dolouroux. Prog Neurosurg Surg. 1976; 7: 180–200

30 Miles JB. Surgical procedures for the relief of pain. In: Williams NE, Wilson H (eds) Pain & its management, Section 112. New York: Pergamon Press, 1983, pp. 89–98

31 Lipton S. Acupuncture for pain relief. In: Acupuncture in medicine. Volume 2, 1988, 26–28

32 Kenyon J. Acupuncture in Pain Relief. In: Lipton S, (ed.) Persistent pain, modern methods of treatment. Volume 2: Academic Press, 1979, pp. 203–222

33 Melzack R, Wall PD. Pain mechanisms: A new theory. Science 1965; 150: 971–979

34 Shealy CN, Mortimer JT, Reswick RJ. Electrical inhibition of pain by stimulation of the dorsal column: Preliminary clinical report. Anaesth Analgesia 1967; 46: 489–491

35 Woolf CJ. Segmental Afferent fibre induced analgesia: Transcutaneous Electrical nerve stimulation (TENS). In: Wall PD, Melzack R, eds. Textbook of pain, 2nd edn. Edinburgh: Churchill Livingstone, 1989, pp. 889–896

36 Miles JB. Assessment for dorsal column stimulation. Proceedings of the combined Meeting of Scandinavian Pain Society and the Intractable Pain Society, Oslo, April 1989

37 Krainick J-U, Thoden U. Pain reduction in amputees by long-term spinal cord stimulation. J Neurosurg 1980; 52: 346–350

38 Meyerson B. Long term treatment by dorsal column stimulation. Proceedings of the combined meeting of Scandinavian Pain Society and the Intractable Pain Society, Oslo, April 1989

39 Forgas I. Mass hysteria during Mass in Mass. Br Med J 1991; 302: 1087
40 Miles JB, Wells JCD. Pain and its management. In: Findlay and Owen ed, Surgery of the Spine. In press
41 Rosomoff HL. Non-operative treatment of the failed back syndrome presenting with chronic pain. In: Long D, Decker BC, eds. Current therapy in neurological surgery. 1985, pp. 200–202
42 Cherry DA, Gourlay GK, Cousins MJ, Gannon BJ. A technique for the insertion of an implantable portal system for the long-term epidural administration of opioids in the treatment of cancer pain. Anaesth Intensive Care 1985; 13: 145–152
43 Magora F. Current status of the utilisation of opioids by spinal injection. In: Scherpereel P, Meynadier J, Blond S, eds. The Pain Clinic II. Utrecht: VNV Science Press, 1987, pp. 79–92

British Medical Bulletin (1991) Vol. 47, No. 3, pp. 786
© The British Council 1991

Erratum

Volume 47 No. 2 Breast Disease

Screening for breast cancer pp 400–415
N E Day

In Table 1 (Summary of major controlled trials of breast cancer) on pp 401 of the above paper, in the line beginning WE(15), the figures for Age at entry (years) should read 40–74 *not* 40–47.

Index